You Are Your Own BEST MEDICINE

You Are Your Own BEST MEDICINE

A Doctor's Advice on the Body's Natural Healing Powers

FRÉDÉRIC SALDMANN, M.D.

Translated by Jack Cain

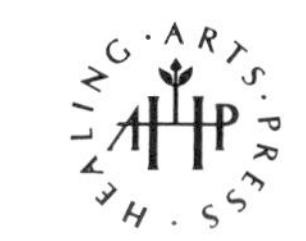

Healing Arts Press
Rochester, Vermont • Toronto, Canada

Healing Arts Press
One Park Street
Rochester, Vermont 05767
www.HealingArtsPress.com

Healing Arts Press is a division of Inner Traditions International

Originally published in French under the title *Le meilleur médicament, c'est vous!* by Éditions Albin Michel
First U.S. edition published in 2016 by Healing Arts Press

Note to the reader: *This book is intended as an informational guide. The remedies, approaches, and techniques described herein are meant to supplement, and not to be a substitute for, professional medical care or treatment. They should not be used to treat a serious ailment without prior consultation with a qualified health care professional.*

Library of Congress Cataloging-in-Publication Data

Saldmann, Frédéric.
[Meilleur médicament c'est vous! English]
You are your own best medicine : a doctors advice on the bodys natural healing powers / Frédéric Saldmann, M.D. ; translated by Jack Cain. — First U.S. edition.
pages cm
Includes bibliographical references and index.
ISBN 978-1-62055-429-6 (paperback) — ISBN 978-1-62055-430-2 (e-book)
1. Health. 2. Health behavior. 3. Families—Health and hygiene. 4. Medicine, Preventive. I. Title.
RA773.S2513 2016
613—dc23
2015011605

Printed and bound in the United States by Versa Press, Inc.

10 9 8 7 6 5 4 3 2 1

Text design and layout by Virginia Scott Bowman
This book was typeset in Garamond Premier Pro and Gill Sans with Helvetica Neue used as the display typeface

For Marine

CONTENTS

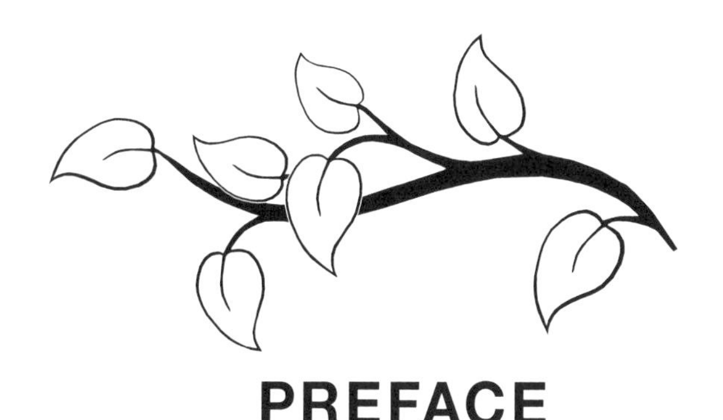

PREFACE

An apple a day keeps the doctor away . . . as long as you have good aim!

WINSTON CHURCHILL

In everyone's eyes my role as a doctor is clearly defined: I listen, I examine, I arrive at a diagnosis, and I prescribe. This is the very essence of my job. However, I have the impression that I don't always meet my patients' deepest needs. In fact, I'm surprised by the number of patients who come back to see me regularly, either to renew a prescription or for some new pathology that is similar to the previous one. With time I've gotten used to always seeing the same faces in my waiting room. Over the years my patients and I have gotten to know each other quite well, establishing a kind of three-way relationship: the doctor, the patient, and the illness. We catch up on each other's news, we worry, we calm down, and we decide to see each other again. Each of us settles into our routine. All is well. But not really—because we can do better with a simple method. The human brain and body in fact have very strong powers available that are almost never used. These powers only need to be activated in order to effectively treat a considerable number of symptoms and illnesses. The effect is double; by correcting the cause and not the effect, you reduce recurrences and you build real fortifications against illness. In our depths we have our own medicines that can be used to heal us, but we don't use them. We are our own medicine, but we don't know it.

By writing this book my intention is to deliver to you the prescription that I would never have dared write for you in an office visit and provide you with a method for being in better health and healing yourself. Let's take a very simple example. Treatments for high cholesterol, type 2 diabetes, and high blood pressure are used by millions of patients. Every day these individuals take tablets that are supposed to protect them from cardiovascular disease. However, statistics clearly show that these pills are not some magic potion. Yes, they lower the risks a little, sometimes with troublesome side effects, but they do not treat the cause. By modifying a few parameters, you can often do without the treatment and correct the problem. In fact, 30 percent fewer calories means 20 percent more life expectancy! Reducing your weight, improving your eating, and engaging in regular physical activity can change everything. One number is enough to understand how basic all this is: thirty minutes of exercise every day reduces the risk of cancer, Alzheimer's, and cardiovascular disease by 40 percent.

And that's not all. On your own and using natural methods, you can protect yourself from and heal numerous illnesses. The human organism is a precision machine that needs perfect balance in order to function without breaking down. Nutrition is a key element. Just imagine putting diesel fuel in a car made for gasoline, and you will have a picture of the damage caused by a fuel that is unbalanced or too rich. There is another topic that I will address in this book even if it means that I'll be out of work one day. I'm talking about all those illnesses that get better quite well on their own without a doctor's help and for which medicines are useless or even dangerous, as is the case with viral sore throats and the flu. When a treatment is prescribed for such an illness, you have the impression that it is contributing to the healing, when in fact it does nothing of the kind. Without medication the result would have been the same.

Throughout your whole life the body is constantly renewing itself.

Every second twenty million cells split into two cells to replace those that are no longer serviceable. The purpose is to make new, identical cells to replace dead cells. Copy errors during this process of cell division are what leads to cancer. Therefore, it is essential that the organism function in an environment that is likely to reduce copy errors as much as possible. These errors have a tendency to increase with age because the immune system doesn't do as good a job at cleaning up. We could mention the example of smoking, which increases the risk of cell mutation in the lungs, throat, and bladder. Stress and lack of sleep or exercise also are obstacles to effective cellular repair.

It is clearly essential to embark on a program of first-line preventive measures in relation to numerous problems so that we correct the causes and not the effects. Clearly, when it comes to your health, you need to be not just a coworker but an active entrepreneur. In this book I will be giving you keys that will allow you to take back control of your own health and pull together the areas that make it up: what you eat, weight, allergies, sleep, moving about, sexuality, stress, growing old. If I were to compare my book to a tool, I would choose the Swiss army knife; it's multipurpose and lets you address all situations in an immediate and practical way. It is not a matter of substituting these suggestions for your personal physician. I ask you to get your doctor's consent before following the advice offered in this book. But I hope that my suggestions will show you how to make faster progress through illnesses and better protect yourself with the means at your disposal. My ambition is to help you live a long life in good health.

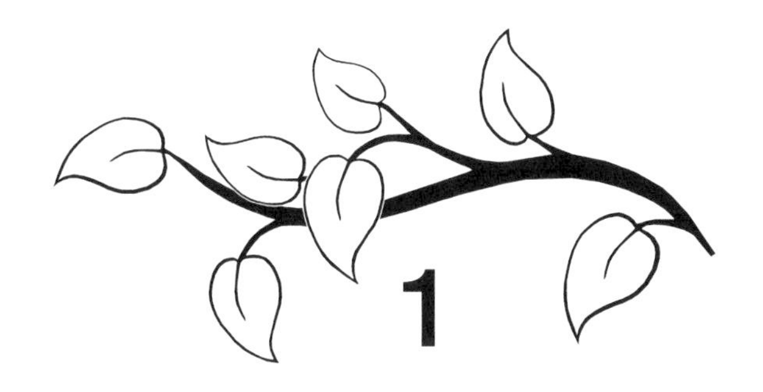

1

TAKING OFF EXCESS WEIGHT

One thing that's even more difficult than sticking to a diet is not imposing it on others.

Marcel Proust

The figures are alarming. In the United States more than one-third of all adults are overweight. According to the WHO being overweight or obese affects 1.4 billion people in the world. That's one person in five. Besides the problem that it causes for public health, excess weight is also a major health risk. It opens the door to both the little daily inconveniences of life such as backache and knee trouble and also serious illnesses such as cancer, cardiovascular disease, or diabetes. Unlike a toothache, which you feel right away, excess weight steadily destroys the body in silence. It's the classic image of someone leading the good life, depriving himself of nothing, and whose life ends abruptly one day, all too quickly and all too terribly. The enormous success of diets—from the most serious to the most weird—shows that many of us wish to lose weight. However, we mustn't cover up the fact that most people who have followed a diet put back all the weight they had lost, or even more, within two years. As a nutritionist I can assure you that the best thing to do to lose weight is to control what you eat while still enjoying eating.

Body Mass Index

To determine if you are overweight, you just need to calculate your BMI (Body Mass Index). Take your weight in pounds divided by your height squared (height times height) in inches and multiply by 703. Or take your weight in kilograms divided by your height squared in meters. If the resulting figure is between 18 and 25, your weight is normal. Above 25 is considered to be overweight, and from 30 up we're into obesity. This index is recognized internationally as a reliable criterion and gets around the assertions of people who say they're not really overweight but just have a heavy bone structure.

APPETITE SUPPRESSORS THAT COMBINE PLEASURE AND EFFECTIVENESS

It's not a secret: to lose weight you have to eat less. The difficulty then is to decrease your appetite. There are two solutions. Either you accept being hungry, and you suffer the first days patiently knowing that the effect will gradually decrease. But that requires great strength of character to resist all those temptations that are always close by! Or you adopt some measures for staying the course, and you quietly get used to a reduced daily caloric intake. Here are some hunger-breaking ideas that you will soon see are very effective.

Virtuous 100 Percent Dark Chocolate

If you are subject to impulse eating that you don't manage to control, do this little exercise—it's quite simple. When you're about to dig into something greasy, sweet, or salty and put on two pounds in five minutes, crunch down two to four squares of 100 percent dark chocolate and simply decide that you will let yourself loose right after that. You're going to see—the result is immediate. Ingesting dark chocolate brings the impulse to eat to a brutal halt without frustration and without pain.

Recent scientific studies have validated this mechanism—a mechanism that is physiological and not psychological as you might think at first glance. Dutch researchers had volunteers either inhale the scent of dark chocolate or swallow 30 grams (1 ounce) of dark chocolate. They noted a significant appetite decrease following ingestion, and more importantly, they detected certain hormonal factors in the blood, such as ghrelin. Ghrelin is a hormone known for its role in the activation of appetite. Its level increases in a subject who is hungry just before a meal and decreases after the meal. The researchers thus noted that the ingestion of 30 grams of dark chocolate (about one ounce) induced a sharp decrease in ghrelin along with the disappearance of appetite.

And the positive effects of dark chocolate don't stop there. A recent study by Dr. Beatrice Golomb in the United States has very unexpectedly shown that those who regularly eat dark chocolate were thinner than those who didn't eat any dark chocolate. It seems very paradoxical; in spite of having 540 calories per 100 grams (about 3.5 ounces), dark chocolate causes weight loss beyond its appetite-reducing effect. The researchers therefore realized that the BMI of dark-chocolate consumers was lower than that of nonconsumers. The experiments were conducted with one thousand men and women having an average age of fifty-seven. It was found that a maximum effect was obtained with a moderate daily intake of about 30 grams of dark chocolate and not with a large weekly or monthly intake. For the time being the researchers have simply taken note of the effect without exactly understanding the underlying physiological mechanisms. It is possible however that the chocolate acts by reducing stress, which contributes to lowering the impulse to eat. Also, chocolate is known for its concentration of polyphenols, molecules with antioxidant properties. In fact, a German study conducted by Dr. Dirk Taubert at the University Hospital of Cologne found that the regular consumption of two squares of dark chocolate a day led to a lowering of blood pressure, with the first number (systolic pressure) coming down by up to three points and the second number (diastolic pressure) by up to two points. Chocolate also increases the flexibility of our arteries through an effect on the viscosity of the blood.

Similarly, we might offer here a further explanation of the famous "French paradox" according to which the French have half as many heart attacks as Americans. This fact is not only linked to the red wine that is taken with every meal but also to dark chocolate. In fact, the French are the greatest consumers of dark chocolate on the planet—six times more than other countries.

It's very easy to find chocolate in supermarkets, but don't make any concessions. I really did say 100 percent chocolate and not 85 percent or 90 percent because the result is not the same. You can keep these precious bars at the office, at home, or in your purse. As soon as you feel the urge, crunch down a few squares . . . in moderation.

The Mysterious Powers of Saffron

Saffron is a spice that originally was extracted from a plant: *Crocus sativus.* For a long time now, there have been stories about its natural appetite-breaking power. And sometimes real facts can be hiding behind such stories. This is what a French research team has recently shown. It seems that saffron has an antisnacking effect and reduces hunger to a significant degree. Snacking is connected to uncontrolled behavior in relation to food, and it predisposes people to excess weight and obesity. The two-month study conducted with sixty women was divided into two groups—one group taking a saffron supplement and the other a placebo. The daily dose of saffron contained in the capsule was 176.5 milligrams. The results showed that the sensation of lack of hunger contributed to reducing the weight-gaining factors. You can use saffron to garnish almost any of your daily dishes: pasta, rice, vegetables, meat, or fish. It does not interfere with the taste of the food—on the contrary, it enhances it. And what's more, it adds a nice color.

Keeping Well Hydrated

I also recommend drinking lots of water during meals, contrary to certain popular ideas. Drinking lots of water is essential for avoiding sudden tiredness, and it is natural that one thinks of drinking during meals. Water also acts as an appetite regulator. Always remember to have two big glasses of water before a social gathering with drinks and snacks. Doing so helps you avoid quenching your thirst with alcoholic drinks and stuffing yourself with French pastries. In the same way beginning a meal by having a big glass of water helps you keep your appetite in check. Besides, all home-entertaining guides recommend filling everyone's water glass before inviting guests to the table.

Your Watch: A Natural Policeman

There are several ways to stop eating. Either you feel that your stomach is so full it will burst from the food you've consumed, which, let's agree, is *not* the most pleasant way—or a sensation that comes about quite differently can take place. If you get in the habit of taking a break for five minutes in the midst of eating your food, before taking second helpings or between each course, a sensation of feeling full will take place naturally. Those precious five minutes allow the satiety center in the brain to be stimulated and set in motion. By practicing these five-minute pauses for a month, you will see that your satiety center, which was asleep, becomes reeducated and starts working marvelously well in its role as an appetite regulator. Without knowing it many restaurant owners adapt to this phenomenon. Using the pretext that their desserts take a long time to prepare or that they might run out of them, they have the waiters take the dessert order at the beginning of the meal. And they're right because you've all had that experience—when the dessert takes too long to appear, you are no longer hungry and will quite readily cancel it.

Egg White: An Unrivalled Hunger Breaker

Proteins, which can come from animal or vegetable sources, are essential components of the cells of the body. Proteins provide our body with azote, an element that it cannot function without. This shows the crucial importance these molecules have for our body. Proteins are present in our daily food: meat, fish, eggs, dairy products, starches, and grains. They have a double advantage; they are very nutritious while also having a low level of calories, which is why they've been successfully worked into certain diets.

Egg white is certainly the star protein-based appetite breaker. With only forty-four calories per 100 grams, egg white is really good at making you feel full. It contains no fat, zero cholesterol, and can be eaten in several forms: hard-boiled egg whites (without the yolk), white omelets, or scrambled egg whites, which can be easily mixed with fresh herbs and tomatoes. You can feel comfortably full for several hours, thus warding off snacking and destabilizing eating binges. Having two hard-boiled egg whites before a socializing snack time helps you avoid diving into the chips and peanuts, even one handful of which represents a real calorie deluge. Scientific research has shown that, given equal amounts of calories, you feel satisfied longer after a meal rich in protein than after a meal rich in carbohydrates and lipids. Eating protein sends an appetite-breaking message to hunger control centers.

Foods Rich in Protein

- White or red meat
- Eggs
- Fish
- Nuts and legumes (almonds, peanuts, lentils, white beans)
- Milk products (yogurt, cheese)

THE MYSTERIES OF CHILIES AND PEPPER

Chilies

Many of you at one time or another may have fallen victim to the experience of downing a hot chili pepper that you didn't notice on your plate. The result is immediate: thirst that won't go away, a really strong sense of heat, and profuse sweating. A team of researchers at the David Geffen School of Medicine in Los Angeles looked at this issue and wondered if there might be a connection between eating chilies and one's weight. Could there really be an effect of the chili burning up fat? These scientists, intrigued by the phenomenon, tested the effect of chilies on a group of volunteers. They began with the hypothesis that chilies could lead to an expenditure of energy and speed up the metabolism. The study showed an increase in thermogenesis (temperature) following the meal, as well as an increase in the oxidation of fat. Another study conducted in Baton Rouge, Louisiana, measured the caloric effect of consuming a chili pepper, which they found amounted to about fifty calories a day, a rather modest amount.

Pepper and Salt: The Brake and the Accelerator

The presence of salt is invisible in food and does constitute a threat to health if consumed in excess. The majority of scientists have sounded an alarm about this. Its link to high blood pressure, cardiovascular disease, an increased occurrence of stomach cancer, and osteoporosis is now clear. More recently, research at the Yale School of Medicine has brought to light a possible connection to autoimmune diseases such as MS (multiple sclerosis). In practice, salt attacks the organism on all fronts, whether it's the arteries or certain cancers that are targeted. It is important to also stress that salt is a very good appetite stimulator; this is why snacks such as peanuts and almonds are salted. For those who want to control their weight, salt is not an ally.

How do you determine if your daily salt intake is excessive? It's not at all easy. No one is going to be able to weigh the salt ingested in one day. Reaching for your calculator to find out how much salt is in that slice of ham or some prepared dish is not practical. Adding up the salt intake in twenty-four hours is like a Chinese puzzle. What you need to do is apply common sense. I advise never putting salt on the table and, even more important, never adding salt before tasting. Getting in the habit of cooking without salt is also a good technique. Try asking for a dish without salt when in a restaurant. This is also a good way to find out if the dish is prepared ahead of time or only when ordered. When you first try this, you will find the dishes dull and tasteless. That lasts about two weeks. Your appetite will decrease sharply. Gradually, you will bring your threshold of saltiness to the brain level. To understand what is happening, it's as if you were in the habit of having your coffee without sugar. If someone adds a lump of sugar, you won't be able to drink it—you'll find it disgusting. The whole spectrum of eating works the same way. That little square of chocolate that you carry around—you won't be able to stand it when it's milk chocolate—you'll want it as dark as possible. You have changed. Your tastes are no longer the same. You don't follow your usual diet anymore; now you have other tastes that you enjoy. With salt you can play the game the same way. By getting used to eating low salt or no salt, you will no longer be able to stand a dish with too much salt. You've won your game. You are protecting your arteries, and your risk of stomach cancer is much lower. And the cherry on the cake is that your appetite is much easier to control.

The fact is we spontaneously use too much salt. The right reflex then is to get used to eating a minimum of salt. A good way to do this is to substitute pepper for salt. Pepper comes in several colors: gray, which only exists in ground form, green, black, and white. These colors generally correspond to various stages of maturity at the time of harvesting the peppercorns. I am deliberately setting aside pink pepper, which should be eaten sparingly because it can have toxic issues (being related to poison ivy) capable of causing headaches, breathing difficulties, diarrhea, or hemorrhoids. If you're really a fan of pink pepper, you should use only a few of the berries in one dish, no more.

You need to know that commercially available pepper is very often initially treated with radiation. Most often, in the countries where it is produced, spices are dried on the ground and contain a lot of bacteria. It is frequently the case that a million bacteria are found in pepper, including salmonella. However, there is no need to panic; the radiation allows the product to be sterilized and consumed with no anxiety. It involves a technique that kills the bacteria in the food and poses no health risk.

Pepper turns out to be an interesting weight-loss ally. It has a variety of properties. It supports a reduction in appetite and facilitates digestion by reducing gas. New properties of this spice are being discovered every day. For example, pepper burns off fat and inhibits adipogenesis (the formation of reserves of fat). Recent studies have been conducted to analyze these surprising functions. Dr. K. J. Kim of Korea has shown that pepper has a weight-loss effect on mice. Other studies have shown an effect in lowering cholesterol. A Canadian team working under Dr. M. Yoshioka studied the effect of red pepper in Japanese women having meals that were especially rich in fat and sugar. They observed that adding pepper increased energy expenditure so that more calories were burned off, producing a sensation of increased body heat. The same effects were observed in men by a team of Japanese researchers working with Dr. Yoshioka, who noticed this same increase of energy expenditure.

DESSERTS THAT MAKE YOU THIN

Dr. Daniela Jakubowicz and her team of Israeli researchers have just erased a taboo by showing that having a dessert at breakfast can contribute more effectively to weight loss. With overweight subjects they observed that those who had a good breakfast accompanied by dessert had much better results in following a diet than those who didn't have a dessert. The group that didn't have dessert lost out twice—because their diet didn't go as well either. Those who had dessert were less subject to cravings and had no desire for sweets during the course of the day. The scientists backed this up with an explanation of the phenomenon. The morning dessert acts to reduce the production of ghrelin, the hormone that produces the feeling of hunger. People who begin their morning with the "super-forbidden"—that is, dessert—get their sugar hit first thing. According to this amazing team of researchers who worked with

193 overweight subjects, the morning dessert will then regulate the sensation of hunger for the whole day.

To stay in shape it's clear that it's better to skip dessert at every meal. It's often difficult when you're sitting down with others and everyone is having one or when the restaurant you're in has a stunning dessert menu! I suggest you have a green tea instead of dessert. Then you won't have an empty plate in front of you as you enviously watch your neighbors. But it's not only that. A team of researchers at Lund University in Malmö, Sweden, has just shown that choosing green tea after the end of the meal will extend your feeling full by two hours.

THE JOY OF KEEPING YOUR WEIGHT IN CHECK

Beware of Ready-to-Eat Light Dishes

Let's be frank: it's often disappointing to buy a light meal that is vacuum-sealed or frozen. Although the photos on the packaging look appetizing and the calorie count specified is reassuring, the frustration appears once it's on your plate. The consumer has the impression of being punished seeing the pitifully meager portion on the plate. "Eat less to weigh less" isn't working. Ridiculously small portions at mealtime lead to uncontrollable impulses to eat during the day. Recently, a little girl in a British school created a blog that caused quite a stir. She simply photographed what she was served in the cafeteria and calculated how many mouthfuls each dish represented.

I have tried this out with several suggested slimming dishes. On the average, within three or four mouthfuls, the meal is over. And if, on top of that, the dish was well prepared and tasty, the frustration is even worse. You have just eaten the amount required to set loose an immense appetite that will be impossible to control.

In order to arrive at the point of feeling full, you need to take into account both physiological and psychological factors. Psychological because, if you consume a large volume of food, the impression of being satisfied is better, and physiological because if the quantity is just right, the baroreceptors that are sensitive to pressure on the inner wall of the stomach will be stimulated, giving rise to an agreeable sensation of feeling full. Certain foods have the capacity to add bulk while adding a very low level of calories: for example, mushrooms (14 calories in 3.5 ounces), tomatoes (21 calories in 3.5 ounces), or even 3.5 ounces of steamed potatoes, which only amounts to 85 calories. A mixed salad made up of these foods, served in a huge salad bowl and garnished with herbs and a touch of balsamic vinegar represents a limited caloric intake and will form the basis of an excellent sensation of feeling full.

Savor the Present Moment

As you are having your first coffee of the day, you are already thinking of the day ahead, projecting yourself into the future while forgetting the present. You're no longer even aware of what you are drinking. This is the moment when you need to close your eyes, concentrate on the coffee's aroma, on the just-right temperature of the water, and the marvelous scent that rises up from the cup. If things are not perfect, you can improve them and create a more pleasant environment. A few examples might be to change the brand of coffee, come to understand the subtle differences in the taste of various substances, choose a good mineral water, adjust the temperature, opt for an improved preparation method, or choose a fine porcelain cup with a thin rim. Learn to build for yourself a new world of pleasure and enjoyment that is just for you. While costing you very little, you will discover subtle and delicate impressions. You need to continue to learn to appreciate them. Concentrating on what you're doing—on the present moment only—allows you to come back to yourself and to be more open to pleasure. What is true for a cup of coffee is also true for many other moments in life. It's a question of focusing on the now and of knowing how to select those small details that add to a feeling of well-being. It's also an excellent way to learn how to lose weight effortlessly. If you swallow your food mechanically while thinking of something else, you risk eating too much. In contrast, it's possible for you to know, with each mouthful, why it is that you want the next mouthful, and in this way you will regulate your weight-loss curve. There's nothing more heartbreaking—and bad for the health—than taking in calories and putting on pounds with dishes that really weren't worth the price they cost in added weight.

LITERATURE

Aldemir, M., E. Okulu, S. Neselioglu, et al. "Pistachio diet improves erectile function parameters and serum lipid profiles in patients with erectile dysfunction." *International Journal of Impotence Research* 23(1) (2011): 32–38.

Al-Dujaili, E., and N. Smail. "Pomegranate juice intake enhances salivary testosterone levels and improves mood and well being in healthy men and women." *Endocrine Abstracts* 28 (2012): 313.

Dreher, M. L. "Pistachio nuts: Composition and potential health benefits." *Nutrition Reviews* 70(4): 234–40.

Freedman, N. D., Y. Park, C. C. Abnet, et al. "Association of coffee drinking with total and cause-specific mortality." *New England Journal of Medicine* 366(20) (2012): 1891–1904.

Galgani, J. E., and E. Ravussin. "Effect of dihydrocapsiate on resting metabolic rate in humans." *American Journal of Clinical Nutrition* 95(5) (2010): 1089–93.

Galgut, J. M., and S. A. Ali. "Effect and mechanism of action of resveratrol: A novel melanolytic compound from the peanut skin of *Arachis hypogaea*." *Journal of Receptors and Signal Transduction Research* 31(5) (2011): 374–80.

Gebauer, S. K., S. G. West, C. D. Kay, et al. "Effects of pistachios on cardiovascular disease risk factors and potential mechanisms of action: A dose-response study." *American Journal of Clinical Nutrition* 99(3) (2008): 651–59.

Golomb, A. B., S. Koperski, and H. L. White. "Association between more frequent chocolate consumption and lower body mass index." *Archives of Internal Medicine* 172(6) (2012): 519–21.

Gout, B., C. Bourges, and S. Paineau-Dubreuil. "Satiereal, a *Crocus sativus* L. extract, reduces snacking and increases satiety in a randomized placebo-controlled study of mildly overweight, healthy women." *Nutritional Research* 30(5) (2010): 305–13.

Jakubowicz, D., O. Froy, J. Wainstein, and M. Boaz. "Meal timing and composition influence ghrelin levels, appetite scores and weight loss maintenance in overweight and obese adults." *Steroids* 77(4) (2012): 323–31.

Jeyaraj, D., S. M. Haldar, X. Wan, et al. "Circadian rhythms govern cardiac repolarization and arrhythmogenesis." *Nature* 483(7387) (2012): 96–99.

Jeyaraj, D., F. A. Scheer, J. A. Ripperger, et al. "Klf15 orchestrates circadian nitrogen homeostasis." *Cell Metabolism* 15(3) (2012): 311–26.

Kim, K. J., M. S. Lee, K. Jo, and J. K. Hwang. "Piperidine alkaloids from *Piper retrofractum* Vahl. protect against high-fat diet induced obesity by regulating lipid metabolism and activating AMP-activated protein kinase." *Biochemical and Biophysical Research Communications* 411(1) (2011): 219–25.

Kleinewietfeld, M., A. Manzel, J. Titze, et al. "Sodium chloride drives autoimmune disease by the induction of pathogenic TH17 cells." *Nature* 496(7446) (2013): 518–22.

Kris-Etherton, P. M., F. B. Hu, E. Ros, and J. Sabaté. "The role of tree nuts and peanuts in the prevention of coronary heart disease: Multiple potential mechanisms." *Journal of Nutrition* 138(9) (2008): 1746S–51S.

Lee, T. A., Z. Li, A. Zerlin, and D. Heber. "Effects of dihydrocapsiate on adaptive and diet-induced thermogenesis with a high protein very low calorie diet: A randomized control trial." *Nutrition & Metabolism* (London) 7(78) (2010): doi:10.1186/1743-7075-7-78.

Liu, Y., V. R. Yadev, B. B. Aggarwal, and M. G. Nair. "Inhibitory effects of black pepper (*Piper nigrum*) extracts and compounds on human tumor cell proliferation, cyclooxygenase enzymes, lipid peroxidation and nuclear transcription factor-kappa-B." *Natural Product Communications* 5(8) (2010): 1253–57.

Massolt, E. T., P. M. van Haard, J. F. Rehfeld, et al. "Appetite suppression through smelling of dark chocolate correlates with changes in ghrelin in young women." *Regulatory Peptides* 161(1–3) (2010): 81–86.

Ogden, C. L., M. D. Carroll, B. K. Kit, and K. M. Flegal. "Prevalence of childhood and adult obesity in the United States, 2011–2012." *JAMA* 311(8) (2014): 806–14.

Park, U. H., H. S. Jeong, E. Y. Jo, et al. "Piperine, a component of black pepper, inhibits adipogenesis by antagonizing PPARγ activity in 3T3-L1 cells." *Journal of Agriculture and Food Chemistry* 60(15) (2012): 3853–60.

Taubert, D., R. Roesen, C. Lehmann, et al. "Effects of low habitual cocoa intake on blood pressure and bioactive nitric oxide: a randomized controlled trial." *JAMA* 298(1) (2007): 49–60.

Turski, M. P., P. Kamiński, W. Zgrajka, et al. "Potato—an important source of nutritional kynurenic acid." *Plant Foods for Human Nutrition* 67(1) (2012): 17–23.

Yoshioka, M., K. Lim, S. Kikuzato, et al. "Effects of red-pepper diet on the energy metabolism in men." *Journal of Nutritional Science and Vitaminology* (Tokyo) 41(6) (1995): 647–56.

Yoshioka, M., S. St-Pierre, M. Suzuki, and A. Tremblay. "Effects of red-pepper added to high-fat and high-carbohydrate meals on energy metabolism and substrate utilization in Japanese women." *British Journal of Nutrition* 80(6) (1998): 503–10.

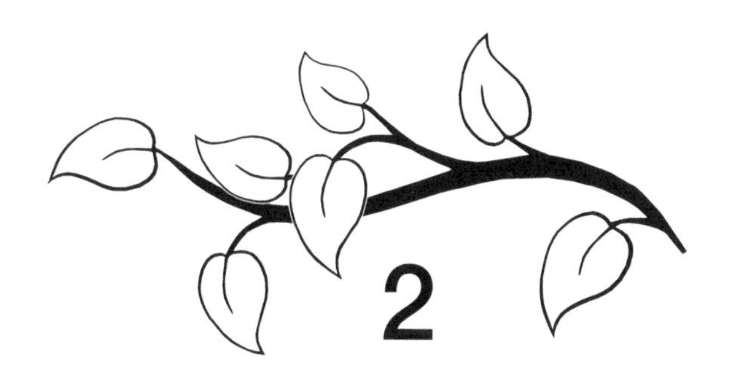

2

GETTING YOUR BODY MOVING

> *All mankind is divided into three classes: those that are immovable, those that are movable, and those that move.*
>
> Benjamin Franklin

Now that you've jettisoned some conventional wisdom, we need to control your weight in order to give your organism a boost and get your energy level reading *full.* Our lives are stressful and sedentary so this isn't always easy. To do it there's just one secret: move! Physical activity is just as essential as brushing your teeth. In fact, regular activity can reduce the general mortality rate by 38 percent, with an even greater effect on certain illnesses (cardiovascular diseases for example). It also helps you fight obesity and aging. For the bolder ones among you, a complementary and quite surprising way of controlling your weight and making your organism more youthful is the practice of fasting, which is discussed a bit later.

THE BENEFITS OF PHYSICAL ACTIVITY

Dangers of a Sedentary Lifestyle

It's an established fact: we consume too many calories every day, and a sedentary lifestyle can't deal with it. In France a man consumes an average of 2500 calories a day and a woman 2200 calories. According to the Dietary Guidelines for Americans 2010, a national survey indicated that men in the United States consume an average of 2,640 daily calories and women 1,785 daily calories. In contrast, it has been observed that, on the island of Okinawa in Japan, famous for its record numbers of one-hundred-year-olds, the inhabitants consume an average of six hundred calories less than the rest of the population. When you realize that an excess of just one hundred calories per day means six pounds more on the scales at the end of the year, you can see why this is so important. But be careful: being in good health is not just a question of being thin. It's regular physical exercise that will make the difference. In fact, physical activity plays an active role in maintaining weight loss after going on a diet by combating the yo-yo effect. This is a significant advantage when you realize that 95 percent of those who adopt a slimming diet put the weight back on within two years of having followed it.

Another thing to bear in mind is that it's not necessarily what the scales are reading that is important. In fact, muscles are heavier than fat. For two bodies of the same height, the muscled person will weigh in heavier than the one cloaked in fat. The mistake people make is thinking that engaging in sports makes you lose weight. It's just one useful component in a general strategy of taking charge of the health of your body. It is only recently that the true benefit of sports to one's health has been discovered. The latest scientific advances have allowed us to learn the precise effect of physical activity on health, the sports that are suitable to engage in, and at what frequency to do so for optimal effectiveness.

The Prevention of Illness

Regular physical activity is above all effective for the prevention of cardiovascular disease. In order to understand this positive effect, researchers conducted various studies that brought out several levels of activity. When the heart has to make a physical effort, more oxygen is required. To respond to this demand, the heart rate increases in order to produce increased blood flow. The heart provides oxygen to the body in red blood cells. When the heart rate increases, the organism then consumes more oxygen. Oxygen is necessary, but at the same time it acts as a kind of poison in the human body, causing the cells to wear out. It's like a car burning too much gas and not giving you good mileage in the end. By getting your heart gradually used to working at faster rates, you promote a reduction in heart rate when you're resting. This is why athletes have slower heart rates. It has been shown that a slower heart rate is good for health. Staying with the metaphor of the car, you can see that a motor that doesn't turn as fast is more economical.

The Blue Whale: A Particular Idea of Eternity

The blue whale is by far the biggest animal living in our era. It is famous for its longevity, from 80 years on the average and extending to as much as 130 years. It can be more than 30 meters long and weigh up to 180 tons (whereas a dinosaur weighed about 90 tons). What is particularly interesting is the relationship between the weight of the animal and its longevity. It has often been established that the more the size of an animal increases, the greater its chances for longevity. It's the opposite for human bodies: increased weight decreases life span. When we look at the physiology of the whale more closely, we see that its heart beats extremely slowly—eight beats per minute when it is at the surface, and the frequency can fall to four beats per minute when the animal is in the ocean depths.

But don't panic if your heart beats too fast when resting. The average heart rate is around sixty beats per minute. If the rate is too high—we call that *tachycardia*—your doctor will do an examination in order to find the cause. Causes for tachycardia are many. Occasionally, it is provoked by physical exertion, fever, drinking too much alcohol, stress, dehydration, taking stimulants, or hyperthyroid medications. Beyond these causes, which are not cardiac, there are other causes that are purely cardiac, ranging from a cardiac deficiency to a pulmonary embolism. If your doctor concludes that you have none of the above, but in spite of that your heart rate during rest is a bit too high, there is an excellent treatment to slow it down and increase longevity: daily physical exercise for thirty to forty minutes a day, such as a fast walk, biking, or swimming.

Cholesterol

Cholesterol is a fatty substance essential to the organism that takes part in the formation of our cells and the synthesis of certain hormones (including those related to sexual function) and vitamin D. Cholesterol is produced mainly by the liver (about two-thirds of it), and the remainder comes from what we eat.

Since physical activity burns sugar and fat, the levels of sugar and bad cholesterol in the blood will decrease correspondingly, reducing the plaque of atheroma that gradually clogs the arteries and is the underlying cause of strokes—with risk of hemiplegia, heart attacks, or arteritis of the lower limbs. It has been observed that the practice of regular physical exercise reduces the propensity for type 2 diabetes by 60 percent. Lastly, demands that lead to increased blood flow have another beneficial effect related to the heart as a pump. Alongside the coronary arteries, which are there to keep the heart well irrigated, small vessels will gradually form to improve blood flow. An actual parallel pathway develops, thus forming a kind of emergency generator whose presence would be crucial if a blockage were to occur in one of the main conduits. The heart that has been engaged in regular training tires less, is more effective, and protects better against the risk of heart attack.

The beneficial effects of physical activity have also been noted on the reduction in frequency of certain cancers, such as colon cancer, prostate cancer, and breast cancer. However, the most surprising recent discovery concerns Alzheimer's disease. This illness, which continues to increase in frequency, for the moment does not have any medical treatment to halt its fearsome progress. It has been observed however that athletic activity contributes to an improvement in blood circulation to the brain and therefore an improved level of oxygen reaching the brain. Physical exercises are also effective for memory, as are mental exercises. Engaging in sports promotes the production of new neurons, thereby contributing to an improvement in learning and memory. The result has the effect of significantly delaying the onset of this terrible illness.

Where and How to Engage in a Sport

Once the connection between daily physical activity and health has been understood, it's then a question of just doing it. Ah, that's the hard part! How many of us make New Year's resolutions and then don't keep them: a subscription to a health club we never set foot in or an exercise machine for the home that ends up in the far reaches of the basement. The excuses we give ourselves are always the same: I don't have time, when I take some vacation then I'll do it . . . and so on. This strategy of putting things off till tomorrow ends up damaging our health. Therefore, things need to be done immediately. The big question is which sport to practice and how often. If you really don't have time to engage in any specific sport, I recommend that you practice simple, low-cost activities such as a fast walk, biking, or running. The most obvious is no doubt a fast walk, but be careful: you mustn't do it just any old way. For it to be effective, you need to walk 3 kilometers (almost 2 miles) in thirty minutes without stopping. During the first twenty minutes, you burn sugar, which is not the most important thing—even though doing so is always good for your health. The main advantage happens in the following ten or twenty minutes during which you burn off bad fat. This exercise is difficult to practice in the city where you have to stop regularly at red lights or just because the sidewalks are too busy.

Diabetes

Diabetes is a malfunction in the assimilation and regulation of sugar (glucose) brought into the organism through eating. When we eat we absorb sugar, which is the main source of energy that keeps the body functioning. In a normal subject it is insulin produced by the pancreas that looks after distributing the sugar through the body and regulating its level in the blood (glycemic level). The normal glycemic level is between 0.70 and 1.10 g/l. In individuals who are diabetic, the regulation is no longer functional and the blood contains too much sugar (hyperglycemic). There are two kinds of diabetes: type 1 diabetes, called insulin dependent, which is found in young people and in which the body is not creating insulin; and type 2, called insulin nondependent or diabetes mellitus, which is found in older people and in which insulin is produced but is not sufficiently active. Type 2 diabetes is more common (85 percent of diabetics) and is often found in overweight and sedentary subjects.

If you can't bike, run, or do a fast walk, a simple pair of barbells will do and will provide the same beneficial effects. In fact, researchers at the Harvard School of Public Health have recently shown the impact of this practice on health. The results show that with two and a half hours of workout with the arms each week using small barbells, which you can easily find in a mall, subjects lowered by 34 percent their probability of contracting type 2 diabetes (see text box on page 20). The explanation is simple—muscles consume a lot of sugar; the more they are developed, the more sugar you burn.

The Miracle of Stairs

Even if you stubbornly refuse to do any physical activity at all, you can't get off that easily! This is because there is one other simple solution, available to everyone, for engaging in exercise daily with ease—stairs. A team under Dr. Meyer at the University Hospital of Geneva in Switzerland carried out a study to determine if going up and down stairs was really beneficial for one's health. To do that he studied seventy-seven individuals for three months, asking them to go up and down twenty-one flights of stairs every day. The results greatly exceeded the scientific expectancy as to the effectiveness of this practice. Going up and down stairs really takes off weight. The loss of weight observed was an average of 550 grams (1.2 pounds) in the participants accompanied by a decrease in the waistline of 1.5 centimeters (0.6 inches). When you realize the direct connection that exists between cardiovascular disease and your waistline, you can understand the importance of this result. As soon as you start going up or down stairs, the calorie counter starts to move in the right direction: 0.11 calories for each step climbed and 0.05 for each step gone down. Someone who goes up and down stairs for fifteen minutes a day loses 150 calories on the average and, if the exercise is continued for thirty minutes, 300 calories, which is the amount of calories in a croissant. Someone who goes up and down the equivalent of twenty-one floors a day will maintain his weight at 2 kilograms (4.4 pounds) below the initial weight before he began. And even the laziest are rewarded—someone who takes the elevator and comes back down on foot will lose at least one kilogram (2 pounds) per year.

The health benefit of stairs does not end there since this practice is also known to prevent cardiovascular illness. The first study that brought this to light was published in 1953 in the prestigious scientific journal *The Lancet,* but it was ignored. It was a study of bus drivers and ticket takers in the city of London. The red buses of this city are all double-decker. The driver spends his day seated, and the ticket taker goes up and down stairs eight hours a day. The study showed that the ticket takers had half as many cardiovascular illnesses as the drivers because of this daily physical activity. Dr. Morris, who initiated this study, commented that he thought the increase in severity of cardiovascular disease was directly connected to lifestyle.

Subsequently, other scientific studies have enabled us to understand why and how climbing stairs contributes to health. In fact, in individuals who decide not to take elevators and climb stairs instead, a significant decrease in blood pressure has been recorded. It is important to be clear that as you are climbing, the blood pressure goes up, but once you stop, the pressure decreases and stabilizes at a lower level in practitioners of the sport of stair climbing. Given that high blood pressure is a veritable scourge that promotes the onset of illnesses such as myocardial infarction (heart attack) and hemiplegia (paralysis of one side of the body), you can understand the attractiveness of a practice that lowers arterial pressure. In the Swiss study by Dr. Meyer, the participants enjoyed an average benefit of a decrease of 1.8 percent in their blood pressure. This form of exercise also contributed to a 3 percent lower level of cholesterol—the substance that gradually blocks the arteries. Breathing capacity was increased by 6 percent at the end of three months, which is excellent for an improved level of oxygenation of the cells.

Daily physical activity is then an obligation, I would almost say a survival requirement, in order to remain healthy. As I made clear in the introduction, thirty minutes of exercise a day reduces all causes of death by 40 percent, whether it's cardiovascular illnesses, cancer, or Alzheimer's. All this can be accomplished simply by using the stairs in your building or in your office. Do the math. In one day it is not hard to manage twenty-one floors. Increasing your physical and breathing capacity, lowering your blood pressure and cholesterol level, getting rid of fat, and reducing your waistline in a lasting way is the benefit you reap from giving up elevators and escalators. What's at stake is too important for you to lose a single minute before beginning.

FASTING . . . FAST TO STAY YOUNG

In the depths of our cells, there is an astonishing hidden function that allows the organism to become young again, as if it was rejuvenating itself. This power can be awakened by a special way of eating: a periodic fast.

An Ancient Power

It all began thousands of years ago when mankind lived hunter-gatherer existences and faced cold, danger, and periods of famine. The organism then adapted by biologically learning how to cope with a period of lack by fasting naturally from time to time. Our ancestors' human body knew how to draw the fuel it needed for life and good health from fatty tissue, regardless of external conditions. In those former times a man weighing 70 kilos (150 pounds) with a height of 1.7 meters (67 inches) could last forty days by drawing on a fatty reserve of 15 kilos (33 pounds). Certain animals of the polar regions, such as penguins, have kept this resistant ability by fasting for several months in the cold and living on their fatty reserves.

Like a signal reaching us from the distant recesses of time, many religions have perpetuated the tradition of fasting at certain periods of the year, reminding us of this secret power buried inside us.

Depending on the belief system, fasting is presented in various ways. In the Catholic or Orthodox religion, it is part of the concept of penitence in order to come closer to God. Fasting is voluntarily depriving oneself of food. In certain cases the faithful only have a single meal each day; in other cases certain foods are forbidden, such as meat. In the Islamic religion the fast is connected to a period that is for self-questioning and self-improvement. In Judaism there is Yom Kippur, and for the Hindus there is the eleventh day of each lunar cycle. In each of these cases, the fast is part of a spiritual practice to lead the faithful closer to God. These religions show us that fasting is possible and doesn't present any particular problem. It should be mentioned that all the religions exclude ill persons, children, and pregnant women from this practice.

In practice the body has learned over the course of centuries how to adapt perfectly to a lack of food. Our biological substance has been forewarned of this lack, but today we no longer know how to deal with excess. Abundance is an enemy to our health. To make the situation worse, physical exertion, which used to be the main way we nourished ourselves, has become increasingly eroded by our sedentary existence. And yet protective mechanisms slumber in the depths of our cells like a secret treasure entrusted to us by our ancestors. Recent discoveries have now brought to light the fact that periodic fasting could be just what is needed to reactivate these ancient processes.

The Benefits of Fasting

First of all we need to make a distinction between a total fast, which can be a political fast (hunger strike), and a religious or periodic fast. The biological mechanisms invoked by each one are radically different.

The periodic fast consists of voluntarily going without food for a precise time and a predetermined period. During the period of fasting, the subject drinks as much water or noncalorie drinks as desired. *In all cases the person will have to consult his or her family doctor in order to determine if he or she is suited to the practice of fasting.* The fast begins starting from the sixth hour after the last meal, because it is during the subsequent hours that new biological mechanisms come into play.

There are various ways of going about fasting, ranging from sixteen to twenty-four hours of abstinence or, alternatively, every other day, one day a week, or one day of fasting every ten days. It is surprising to realize that the positive effects of periodic fasting are not restricted to just getting rid of excess pounds but are also connected to illnesses that involve inflammation such as rheumatism, allergies, and asthma. The voluntary doing without food for periods ranging from sixteen to twenty-four hours reactivates an ancient biological memory that knew how to manage a lack of food by installing protective mechanisms. What seems very surprising is the difference in what takes place when we compare ordinary calorie reduction—which consists of a daily reduction of food intake—and periodic fasting, which entails a period of doing without food.

The Renewal of Cells

Our body is a factory that never stops. Out of the sixty trillion cells that make up the body, a significant portion are renewed every day. Each cell, such as a red blood cell or a cell in the stomach, has its own replacement cycle. The key point is that the number of cellular mistakes arising from the copying process used in cell replacement increases with age. A faultily copied cell can become a cancer cell that can, in turn, produce other cells with the same anomalies. The older one gets, the greater is the risk of copying errors. This is why a given risk factor will have different impacts at different ages. Comparing a young person of twenty who smokes a pack of cigarettes a day and a subject of seventy who does the same thing, the risk zone is different. The copying mechanisms of the older subject are much more vulnerable.

Many countries have instituted the practice of controlled, periodic fasting, in particular Germany. Medical teams that have been working in this area for several decades highlight a number of phenomena. One aspect is that fasting sets off a slight increase in adrenaline and noradrenaline, which creates increased vigilance, and this takes place after just sixteen hours. The subject does better at concentrating and is mentally more agile. This is certainly a recurrence of what our ancestors experienced in having to hunt in spite of fasting. In addition, the German doctors think that this type of fasting would increase life expectancy as well as resistance to numerous pathologies. They are working from the hypothesis that when the organism contains damaged cells, it takes the easy way out by destroying them and then replacing them, which speeds up aging. During periods of periodic fasting, the organism reacts differently by repairing cells instead of eliminating them. This illustrates a mechanism that conserves energy while at the same time reduces the risk of making a faulty copy of the DNA, especially in subjects who are getting on in years. They have also noticed that the periodic fast leads to a lower blood-sugar level and reduces insulin-resistance factors. Lastly, the researchers noticed that this way of eating also reduces the production of free radicals (unstable oxygen molecules that try to bond with other cells to become stable and in doing so foster the wearing out of our cells, a little like rust), solely based on the reduction of food intake.

In any case the periodic fasts of many religions open up important new ways of thinking for us. The work of Dr. Berrigan of the National Cancer Institute in Bethesda, Maryland, is particularly interesting in the impact that periodic fasting has on the frequency of cancers. This researcher chose mice that have a shortened lifespan because they had been subjected to a system that naturally lowers the frequency of cancer (Protein 53). He found that in the group of mice that had been subjected to one day of fasting per week, the frequency of cancer went down by 20 percent compared to the group that was fed daily. These results bring our attention to biological changes that correspond to the activation of actual systems of cellular repair. The work has highlighted the concept of a weekly frequency in producing significant results.

Proteus anguinus: The Human Fish That Can Go Ten Years without Eating

This is a strange amphibian that has a body 20 to 40 centimeters (7.9 to 15.8 inches) long and weighs 15 to 20 grams (0.5 to 0.7 ounces). It was named the human fish because its skin resembles that of a human. It can attain one hundred years of age, which is unusual for this type of animal, but also, it is able to withstand situations that would normally kill any living being. It can go ten years without eating anything, and it can manage to live for three days without oxygen! Also we need to mention that it knows how to economize; in a normal situation it is only active for five minutes a day. Two French teams have been especially concentrating on its astonishing abilities. It seems that this animal has the faculty of managing its energy reserves perfectly. It knows how to make the best use of energy while producing very few waste products. In all cells, those of man as well as those of this strange fish, there are real little energy stations called mitochondria whose job it is to provide us with energy. The mitochondria output of this animal is exceptional. Using very little oxygen mitochondria supply the ATP (adenosine triphosphate) that permits the chemical reactions that are vital to the organism to take place. A life-sustaining cycle is then set up: using very little fuel very little waste is generated by the organism, which means less clogging of the natural filters provided to eliminate pollutants from the animal's body. The secret of longevity for the human fish lies then in its ability to extract a maximum amount of energy from the smallest intake while producing minimal waste, which would wear out cells prematurely. This little animal is a kind of master at ecology and sustainable development and illustrates just how interesting this perspective is, both societally and scientifically.

The Practice of Fasting

The length and kind of fasting depends on the person. Those suffering from hypoglycemia are not included in this practice because fasting for them could produce sensations of weakness, light-headedness, sweats, or tiredness. Those who have such difficulties know very well that they will not be able to keep going very long without eating. Clearly, each individual case requires a green light from one's doctor before practicing intermittent fasting.

Intermittent fasting usually lasts from sixteen to twenty-four hours. In practice this means, for example, having only one meal a day. In all cases it is very important to either drink lots of water or have drinks that don't add calories. Some people manage twenty-four hours without difficulty, while for others it can be sixteen hours or less. Each person needs to find the cycle that suits best. Some people have only one meal a day but have fruit in the morning. Others find it easy to do without that sandwich, gobbled down in five minutes at noon, and don't even miss it. Contrary to what you might think, choosing a day of the week when you're really busy makes it easier than a day when you're home prowling around the refrigerator. One point I need to bring to your attention is that you need to avoid making the first meal after an intermittent fast a real flood of calories. The way you can avoid this is easy. All you need to do is think ahead and organize the menu for that first meal and then stick to it.

I have been surprised by the stories of many people who practice this intermittent fast. Many noticed an absence of sensations of hunger. They realized that they sat down to eat every day almost mechanically because it was mealtime, but they weren't really hungry. They found that the real sensation of hunger happened much later. A good number of my patients have noticed important benefits of this practice: they feel less tired, think faster, have more energy, their complexion clears, they have fewer headaches, and feel more upbeat. Overall, there are lots of positive sensations accompanied by a feeling of well-being.

Intermittent fasting allows the organism to regenerate and reactivate the mechanisms of cell repair during sleep. It's also a way of slowing down the effects of passing time so you can live longer in better health. After having consulted your doctor, I advise you to try it out and come to your own conclusions about what you experience.

LITERATURE

Albu, J. B., L. K. Heilbronn, D. E. Kelley, et al. "Metabolic changes following a 1-year diet and exercise intervention in patients with type 2 diabetes." *Diabetes* 59(3) (2010): 627–33.

Aldemir, M., E. Okulu, S. Neşelioğlu, et al. "Pistachio diet improves erectile function parameters and serum lipid profiles in patients with erectile dysfunction." *International Journal of Impotence Research* 23(1) (2011): 32–38.

Barrès, R., J. Yan, B. Egan, et al. "Acute exercise remodels promoter methylation in human skeletal muscle." *Cell Metabolism* 15(3) (2012): 405–11.

Benziane, B., M. Björnholm, S. Pirkmajer, et al. "Activation of AMP-activated protein kinase stimulates Na+, K+-ATPase activity in skeletal muscle cells." *Journal of Biological Chemistry* 287(28) (2012): 23451–63.

Berrigan, D., S. N. Perkins, D. C. Haines, and S. D. Hursting. "Adult-onset calorie restriction and fasting delay spontaneous tumorigenesis in p53-deficient mice." *Carcinogenesis* 23(5) (2002): 817–22.

Bonorden, M. J., O. P. Rogozina, C. M. Kluczny, et al. "Intermittent calorie restriction delays prostate tumor detection and increases survival time in TRAMP mice." *Nutrition and Cancer* 61(2) (2009): 265–75.

Cantó, C., L. Q. Jiang, A. S. Deshumukh, et al. "Interdependence of AMPK and SIRT1 for metabolic adaptation to fasting and exercise in skeletal muscle." *Cell Metabolism* 11(3) (2010): 213–19.

Cleary, M. P., and M. E. Grossmann. "The manner in which calories are restricted impacts mammary tumor cancer prevention." *Journal of Carcinogesis* 10 (2011): 21. doi:10.4103/1477-3163.85181.

DECODE Study Group. "Glucose tolerance and cardiovascular mortality: Comparison of fasting and 2-hour diagnostic criteria." *Archives of Internal Medicine* 161(3) (2011): 397–405.

Egan, B., B. P. Carson, P. M. Garcia-Roves, et al. "Exercise intensity-dependent regulation of peroxisome proliferator-activated receptor coactivator-1 mRNA abundance is associated with differential activation of upstream signalling kinases in human skeletal muscle." *Journal of Physiology* 588(10) (2010): 1779–90.

Fusco, S., C. Ripoli, M. V. Podda, et al. "A role for neuronal cAMP responsive-element binding (CREB)-1 in brain responses to calorie restriction." *Proceedings of the National Academy of Sciences* 109(2) (2012): 621–26.

Ganzer, C., and C. Zauderer. "Promoting a brain-healthy lifestyle." *Nursing Older People* 23(7) (2011): 24–27.

Grøntved, A., E. B. Rimm, W. C. Willett, et al. "A prospective study of weight training and the risk of type 2 diabetes mellitus in men." *Archives of Internal Medicine* 172(17) (2012): 1306–12.

Hara, M. R., J. J. Kovacs, E. J. Whalen, et al. "A stress response pathway regulates DNA damage through β2-adrenoreceptors and β-arrestin-1." *Nature* 477(7364) (2011): 349–53.

Harvie, M. N., M. Pegington, M. P. Mattson, et al. "The effects of intermittent or continuous energy restriction on weight loss and metabolic disease risk markers: A randomized trial in young overweight women." *International Journal of Obesity* 35(5) (2011): 714–27.

Heilbronn, L. K., A. E. Civitarese, I. Bogacka, et al. "Glucose tolerance and skeletal muscle gene expression in response to alternate day fasting." *Obesity Research* 13(3) (2005): 574–81.

Heilbronn, L. K., L. de Jonge, M. I. Frisard, et al. "Effect of 6-month calorie restriction on biomarkers of longevity, metabolic adaptation, and oxidative stress in overweight individuals: A randomized controlled trial." *Journal of the American Medical Association* 295(13) (2006): 1539–48.

Heilbronn, L. K., S. R. Smith, C. K. Martin, et al. "Alternate-day fasting in nonobese subjects: Effects on body weight, body composition, and energy metabolism." *American Journal of Clinical Nutrition* 81(1) (2005): 69–73.

Hervant, F., J. Mathieu, and J. Durand. "Behavioural, physiological and metabolic responses to long-term starvation and refeeding in a blind cave-dwelling (*Proteus anguinus*) and a surface-dwelling (*Euproctus asper*) salamander." *Journal of Experimental Biology* 204 (2001): 269–81.

———. "Metabolism and circadian rhythms of the European blind cave salamander *Proteus anguinus* and a facultative cave dweller, the Pyrenean newt (*Euproctus asper*)." *Canadian Journal of Zoology* 78(8) (2000): 1427–32.

Heydari, A. R., A. Unnikrishnan, L. V. Lucente, and A. Richardson. "Caloric restriction and genomic stability." *Nucleic Acids Research* 35(22) (2007): 7485–96.

Ho, A. J., C. A. Raji, J. T. Backer, et al. "The effect of physical activity, education, and body mass index on the aging brain." *Human Brain Mapping* 32(9) (2011): 1371–82.

Johnson, J. B., S. John, and D. R. Laub. "Pretreatment with alternate day modified fast will permit higher dose and frequency of cancer chemotherapy and better cure rates." *Medical Hypotheses* 72(4) (2009): 381–82.

Karbowska, J., and Z. Kochan. "Intermittent fasting up-regulates Fsp27/Cidec gene expression in white adipose tissue." *Nutrition* 28(3) (2012): 294–99.

Katare, R. G., Y. Kakinuma, M. Arikawa, et al. "Chronic intermittent fasting improves the survival following large myocardial ischemia by activation of BDNF/VEGF/PI3K signaling pathway." *Journal of Molecular and Cellular Cardiology* 46(3) (2009): 405–12.

Katzmarzyk, P. T., T. S. Church, C. L. Craig, and C. Bouchard. "Sitting time and mortality from all causes, cardiovascular disease, and cancer." *Medicine and Science in Sports and Exercise* 41(5) (2009): 998–1005.

Katzmarzyk, P. T., and I. M. Lee. "Sedentary behaviour and life expectancy in the USA: A cause-deleted life table analysis." *BMJ Open* 2(4) (2012): doi: 10.1136/bmjopen-2012-000828.

Langdon, K. D., and D. Corbett. "Improved working memory following novel combinations of physical and cognitive activity." *Neurorehabilitation and Neural Repair* 26(5) (2012): 523–32.

Larsen, J. J., F. Dela, M. Kjaer, et al. "The effect of moderate exercise on postprandial glucose homeostasis in NIDDM patients." *Diabetologia* 40(4) (1997): 447–53.

Larsen, J. J., F. Dela, S. Madsbad, and H. Galbo. "The effect of intense exercise on postprandial glucose homeostasis in Type II diabetic patients." *Diabetologia* 42(11) (1999): 1282–92.

Man, D. W., W. W. Tsang, and C. W. Hui-Chan. "Do older t'ai chi practitioners have better attention and memory function?" *Journal of Alternative and Complementary Medicine* 16(12) (2010): 1259–64.

Meyer, P., B. Kayser, M. P. Kossovsky, et al. "Stairs instead of elevators at workplace: cardioprotective effects of a pragmatic intervention." *European Journal of Cardiovascular Prevention and Rehabilitation* 17(5) (2010): 569–75.

Morris, J. N., J. A. Heady, P. A. B. Raffle, et al. "Coronary heart disease and physical activity of work." *The Lancet* 262(6795) (1953): 1053–57.

Netz, Y., T. Dwolatzky, Y. Zinker, et al. "Aerobic fitness and multidomain cognitive function in advanced age." *International Psychogeriatrics* 23(1) (2011): 114–24.

Raffaghello, L., F. Safdie, G. Bianchi, et al. "Fasting and differential chemotherapy protection in patients." *Cell Cycle* 9(22) (2010): 4474–76.

Safdie, F. M., T. Dorff, D. Quinn, et al. "Fasting and cancer treatment in humans: A case series report." *Aging* 1(12) (2009): 988–1007.

Singh, R., D. Lakhanpal, S. Kumar, et al. "Late-onset intermittent fasting dietary restriction as a potential intervention to retard age-associated brain function impairments in male rats." *Age* 34(4) (2012): 917–33.

Tajes, M., J. Gutierrez-Cuesta, J. Folch, et al. "Neuroprotective role of intermittent fasting in senescence-accelerated mice P8 (SAMP8)." *Experimental Gerontology* 45(9) (2010): 702–10.

Takaishi, T., K. Imaeda, T. Tanaka, et al. "A short bout of stair climbing-descending exercise attenuates postprandial hyperglycemia in middle-aged males with impaired glucose tolerance." *Applied Physiology Nutrition and Metabolism* 37(1) (2012): 193–96.

Timmers, S., E. Konings, L. Bilet, et al. "Calorie restriction-like effects of 30 days of resveratrol supplementation on energy metabolism and metabolic profile in obese humans." *Cell Metabolism* 14(5) (2011): 612–22.

Varady, K. A. "Intermittent versus daily calorie restriction: Which diet regimen is more effective for weight loss?" *Obesity Reviews* 12(7) (2011): 593–601.

Voituron, Y., M. de Fraipont, J. Issartel, et al. "Extreme lifespan of the human fish (*Proteus anguinus*): A challenge for ageing mechanisms." *Biology Letters* 7(1) (2011): 105–7.

Wan, R., I. Ahmet, M. Brown, et al. "Cardioprotective effect of intermittent fasting is associated with an elevation of adiponectin levels in rats." *Journal of Nutritional Biochemistry* 21(5) (2010): 413–17.

Zhao, K. Q., A. T. Cowan, R. J. Lee, et al. "Molecular modulation of airway epithelial ciliary response to sneezing." *FASEB Journal* 26(8) (2012): 3178–87.

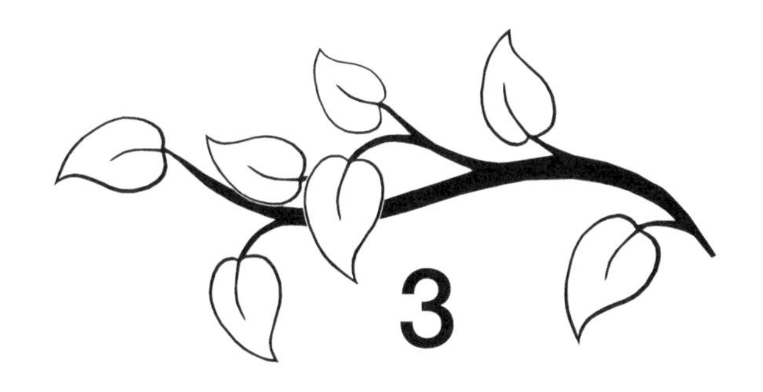

3

IMPROVING YOUR SLEEP

The ideal of calm exists in a sitting cat.

Jules Renard

Sleep is the essential foundation of good health. Physiologically, it allows the organism to regenerate, and psychologically, it helps get rid of tension and unconscious thoughts through the mechanism of dreams. The number of hours of sleep that you need varies from one person to the next, but on the whole, if you are getting under seven hours, you are going short on sleep. Further, a night that is interrupted by frequently waking up will not be as effective as a period of sleeping straight through. In the United States an average of 6.8 hours of sleep per night is reported, according to a 2013 Gallup poll. In France people sleep an average of 7 hours and 13 minutes.* However, sleeping pills continue to be popular; nearly one Frenchman in three and 43 percent of Americans think that they do not get enough sleep. Besides causing trouble concentrating and the unpleasant sensation of brain fog, poor sleep quality engenders a state of chronic fatigue that leads to numerous pathologies of a psychological nature (stress, depression, and the like) or of a physical nature (cardiovascular disease, type 2 diabetes, obesity).

---

*Source: INPES (Institut national de prévention et d'éducation pour la santé [National Institute for Prevention and Health Education]), 2010.

GETTING TO SLEEP

Cherry Juice—A Natural Sleep Inducer

British scientists working under Dr. Glyn Howatson at Northumbria University have recently shown the astonishing effects of cherry juice on falling asleep. Cherry juice acts by increasing the level of melatonin secreted at night and promotes sleep cycles. By drinking only 30 milliliters (a tenth of an ounce) of cherry juice twice a day, volunteers noticed that their time asleep increased by twenty-five minutes after one week. Kiwis also have beneficial effects. As for me, I much prefer having a cherry-kiwi drink to promote a good night's sleep instead of using sleeping pills, which produce poor-quality sleep and a heavy waking up.

Basic Reflexes

Sleep is essential for regenerating your brain. In order to give yourself the best chance of having a good night, you only need to apply a few commonsense rules:

- You need to avoid having too big an evening meal or working out just before going to sleep. Have your evening meal relatively early so that the process of digestion is well underway when you go to bed. You've already seen how poorly you sleep after a late and heavy meal.
- You need to take care that your bedroom is quiet, well ventilated, and especially not too hot. A body temperature that is even slightly too high will disturb your sleep. The ideal temperature for the bedroom—which, as mentioned, needs to be well ventilated—is between 60 and 68 degrees Fahrenheit.
- The hour before sleep should be devoted to activities that are quiet and not stressful. Therefore, it is best to turn off screens

(computers, TV, and smart phones) and to give yourself over to pastimes that promote serenity, like reading, music, or cuddling.

- Also you will find it helpful to always go to bed at the same time every day. By fostering such bedtime rituals, you will get your body used to distinguishing activity time from sleep time.

Lighting

As far as you can, you need to have complete darkness in your bedroom. If that's not possible don't hesitate to buy an eye mask at the drugstore. Researchers at Ohio State University have shown that in hamsters, exposure to artificial light at night promotes depressive behavior. The reason is simple: as with humans, nighttime exposure to light engenders hormonal changes and has an effect on cerebral neurotransmitters. For fifty years now the level of depression has been steadily increasing and can be correlated with the fact that our environment is illuminated more and more with artificial light (screens, signs, billboards). Other studies conducted with hamsters have shown that an increase in states of depression, and often obesity, are linked to light sources that were present during sleep. The final study of this kind on hamsters led to the identification of a specific protein that explains the link between nighttime lighting and depression. Blocking this protein protected hamsters who were exposed to light at night from depression. Be sure to remove all sources of light pollution in your bedroom, even minimal ones such as the points of light from a console, a cell phone being charged, or a TV in sleep mode. You will save on power, and you will awaken full of positive energy in the morning.

Sleep on the Right Side

There is an old proverb that says, "How you make your bed is how you will sleep." This is true literally as well as figuratively. Your state of health will vary depending on whether you sleep on the right side or the left, on a mattress with or without springs, whether or not there's a heated blanket, and whether or not there's a simple night-light in the bedroom. Scientific studies on infants have shown us the direction. Just by having a baby sleep on her back and not on her stomach substantially decreases the incidence of sudden infant death syndrome. Adults, too, need to find out what is the right position for them. It's never too late to get it right!

A chain of British hotels carried out a survey with three thousand of its guests to find out if sleeping on the right side or the left side of the bed had any effect on well-being. The results showed that those who slept on the left side woke up in a better mood, were less stressed, and had a more positive attitude. The results also showed that 25 percent of those surveyed who had spent the night on the left side had a positive outlook on life compared to 18 percent of those who had slept on the right side. Certain behavioral psychologists are studying this issue. They think that when a man sleeps on the left side, he has a protective and realistic character, and when a woman sleeps on the right side, she is more romantic and affectionate. But it is also a question of civilization. In the Chinese culture and in the feng shui approach, spending the night on the right side is to be linked to the masculine yang, which is synonymous with responsibility and action, whereas the left side represents the yin of the feminine and corresponds to receptivity.

Research on finding the right position in bed has led to numerous scientific studies and has led to profound changes in medical recommendations. For decades we wrongly thought that babies should be put to sleep on their stomachs. We thought in fact that this position would avoid choking in the case of reflux. Today things have changed, and doctors recommend to everyone to put babies to sleep on their backs because this position substantially reduces the risk of sudden infant death syndrome. You just need to think of the baby under its covers sinking into too soft a mattress to understand that, in this case, it's the oxygen that's missing. If the infant has a tendency to have reflux, you can just place a big book under the top of the bed to tilt the mattress up a bit. I also recommend that adults who have hiatal hernia with acid reflux be careful not to go to bed too soon after a meal but to wait at least two hours. For those who like watching TV in bed, it's best to use two or three pillows so you are in a semiseated position.

The most astonishing study comes from Dr. Hallberg in Sweden who researched the frequency of cancers in relation to sleeping position. He wondered why certain cancers appeared on one side rather than the other in the human body. He was particularly interested in two kinds of cancer: lung cancer and skin cancer in men and in women. His study revealed that there was a higher incidence of these two cancers in the left side of the body. He was especially surprised by the fact that areas usually little exposed to the sun—known to be a risk factor in melanomas of the skin—paradoxically showed a greater frequency of these cancers: the hips and thighs in women and the trunk of the body in men. He also noticed that this difference between left side and right side and the atypical localization of melanomas was not to be found in Japan.

The Case of the Electric Blanket

Even an object as ordinary as an electric blanket can, in the long run, affect health. Dr. Abel of Wayne State University in Detroit, Michigan, studied the unexpected connections between heating blankets and cancer of the uterus. He found that women who used electric blankets at night for more than twenty years had a higher incidence of cancer of the uterus. The use of these blankets is not common in France but much more frequent in Anglo-Saxon countries. It is clear that the occasional use of these blankets is not dangerous, but repeated use of this kind of heating is not harmless either. For now no cause can be clearly identified to explain this curious phenomenon.

Dr. Hallberg noticed that our mattresses contain metallic springs that can conduct electromagnetic fields, unlike in Japan where sleeping modes are different. Futons are placed directly on the ground and are never made up of metallic structures. Dr. Hallberg and his team of researchers believe that the springs of the bed provide a reception zone for electromagnetic fields to which people are exposed for long periods at night. The researchers then thought that the paradoxically higher frequency of melanoma in the parts of the body identified in their study (the trunk in men and the hips and lower limbs in women) as compared to those body parts exposed to the sun, such as the face, can be explained by exposure at night to electromagnetic fields generated by springs in the mattress.

WAKING UP RIGHT

Early Risers Are Thinner and Happier

A team of British researchers compared two groups of people: a first group who woke up at 7:47 a.m. and a second group who woke up at 10:09 a.m. The study was conducted with one thousand subjects and used two types of measurement: psychological scales to define the level of well-being of the participants and weight and height to evaluate the condition of being overweight. They found that the early risers were in better health, thinner, and happier. The scientists noted as well that the morning people were more willing to have a hearty breakfast that allowed them to maximize their energy reserves and to snack less during the following hours. The internal body clock releases the secretion of certain hormones such as cortisol, which reaches its maximum level every day at 8 a.m. When you realize that cortisol contributes to morning energy, we certainly have the beginning of an explanation.

Wake Up Once

Falling asleep again after turning off the alarm leads to tiredness during the day: this is the conclusion of a study conducted by Dr. Edward Stepanski of Rush University Medical Center in Chicago. Falling asleep again has a counterproductive effect. This is the well-known sensation of being "fuzzy" until late in the morning. The best solution seems to be to wake up with the radio by placing it at some distance from the bed so you don't fall victim to the reflex of just shutting it off and going back to sleep.

Six Ways to Be in Shape on Waking Up

- Avoid an aggressive alarm clock or a radio at full volume.
- Take your time: set your alarm clock fifteen minutes early to avoid rushing.
- Before getting out of bed, stretch like a cat to gently wake up your body: arms, legs, neck, and so on.
- Take a cold shower; it's excellent for body tone.
- Don't skimp on breakfast; it can be suited to your taste—fruit, bread, milk products.
- Practice positive thinking: if your schedule is packed, you can, for example, mentally visualize the end of the day when you'll be getting home to take a nice bath or to be with your children.

Sleeping In Doesn't Help You Catch Up

Sleeping in on the weekend does not allow you to completely recover from tiredness during the week. When you've been burning the candle at both ends several days in a row by sleeping less than six hours a night, you don't reset your counter to zero by sleeping more on Saturday and Sunday.

A team of researchers working with Dr. Alexandros Vgontzas at Penn State University did studies on a group of subjects who were asked to not sleep more than six hours a night for six nights in a row but who then had the chance to sleep ten hours for two nights in a row. After a week with a moderate lack of sleep, the two catch-up nights led to an improved quality of sleep but not of performance. The sleeping in did not eliminate the accumulated fatigue, and the participants had a tendency to be a little clumsy and sleepy Sunday morning, feeling as though they hadn't quite landed. In contrast, it was noted that male sexual performance was restored with the longer night. The researchers highlighted the differences between men and women in relation to sleep. It seems that women benefit more in health from the protective effects of good nights of sleep and that they recuperate more quickly from nights that have been too short.

In general, I advise you to get up one hour later on the weekend, but no more than that, so as not to unbalance your body's sleep pattern. In contrast however, don't hesitate to take a siesta of about twenty minutes after lunch.

SLEEP ENEMIES: SNORING AND APNEA

Snoring

Snoring happens when the palate or the uvula vibrate during sleep from the passage of air. Snoring itself is not dangerous. It can simply disturb the partner's sleep since it produces at least 50 decibels (the equivalent of a human voice). In some cases it can even reach 90 decibels (the noise of a motorbike). Snoring is more likely when overweight, drinking alcoholic beverages, taking sleeping pills or sedatives, with nasal congestion, and with age. In general, before menopause, women are less affected by snoring because of the action of progesterone, which promotes air circulation among other things. Otolaryngology problems also can lead to snoring, such as a simple displacement of the nasal septum or the presence of abnormally enlarged tonsils. One's position in the bed can also increase snoring. Individuals who have a habit of sleeping on their backs snore more. In fact, in this position the tongue is positioned further back, and because of that the air passage is narrower. Since we move around a lot at night, the trick is to stay in the right position to combat snoring.

In practice it is advised to sleep on your stomach and possibly on your side. One known trick you can use is to wear a T-shirt to bed that has a pocket sewn on the back where you can place a tennis ball. This is very effective in maintaining a good posture. The position of the head is also important—using pillows to lengthen the neck helps decrease snoring. Another solution is to tilt the bed up a bit. Finally, if the potential snorer abstains from consuming alcohol or taking tranquillizers before going to bed, he will maximize the chances of his partner getting a good night's sleep.

Sleep Apnea

Things need to be taken more seriously if the snoring is accompanied by sleep apnea. In such cases the health risks are not insignificant. Sleep apnea is characterized by an involuntary cessation of breathing during sleep that extends from ten to thirty seconds and repeats during the night.

Those who are overweight are more liable to have sleep apnea because of the excess fat in the area of the neck that reduces the diameter of the breathing passageways. Independently, it has been observed that the broader the neck, the more likely it is that sleep apnea will occur. The risk starts going up beginning with a neck measurement of 43 centimeters (17 inches) for men and 40 centimeters (16 inches) for women. Individuals who are major consumers of alcohol, drugs, or sleeping pills also push up the risk of sleep apnea.

Sleep apnea wears out the body prematurely. Sleep is essential in the regeneration of body cells. In the case of apnea, the reparative physiological mechanisms are disturbed. The initial symptoms are classic: fatigue during the day, small states of depression, memory problems, frequent drops in energy level, excessive irritability, and headaches.

The most disturbing risk is that of cardiovascular disease provoked by sleep apnea. In fact, the brain is repeatedly exposed to momentary oxygen deficits during the night, which lead to abrupt mini-wakeups that cause an increase in arterial blood pressure and cardiac rhythm. Individuals who have sleep apnea are more at risk for high blood pressure, heart attacks, strokes, and cardiac arrhythmia. In the case of severe apnea, there is an increased risk of dying abruptly during sleep. In the same way the risks during anesthesia are also greater.

It is therefore essential to know whether or not snoring is accompanied by sleep apnea. Sometimes the partner will notice the characteristic pauses in breathing. Awakened by one's snoring neighbor, it is easy to hear the silence associated with sleep apnea in the middle of the night. Sometimes one's attention is caught by an excess of sleepiness during the day or by finding oneself being woken up too often at night. The right response is to consult a medical specialist who can determine the diagnosis of sleep apnea. The overnight examination consists of measuring the frequency and duration of periods of sleep apnea, brain activity, and the level of oxygen in the blood by means of electrodes placed on the body.

Striving to keep the weight off and the practice of physical exercise will clearly contribute to diminishing the risk of sleep apnea. In this regard let's take a look at the work of Brazilian scientists who have been studying the effects of oropharyngeal exercises on patients presenting moderate sleep apnea. They began from the principle that sleep apnea was connected to a loosening in the muscular fibers and that development of a fitness program could make things better. For half an hour a day over a period of three months, the subjects had to rigorously perform several exercises, such as forcefully pressing their tongue into various points on the palate. The results showed an improvement of symptoms compared with a control group who didn't do any daily exercises. If preventive measures don't work, there are various therapeutic means for improving apnea. A doctor can prescribe machines to wear during the night. These machines insufflate air through the nose using a mask. In any case don't ignore sleep apnea—it can be disastrous for your organism.

LITERATURE

Abel, E. L., S. L. Hendrix, G. S. McNeeley, et al. "Use of electric blankets and association with prevalence of endometrial cancer." *European Journal of Cancer Prevention* 16(3) (2007): 243–50.

Bedrosian, T. A., L. K. Fonken, J. C. Walton, et al. "Dim light at night provokes depression-like behaviors and reduces CA1 dendritic spine density in female hamsters." *Psychoneuroendocrinology* 36(7) (2011): 1062–69.

Gregosky, M. J., A. Vertegel, A. Shaporev, and F. A. Treifer. "Tension Tamer: Delivering meditation with objective heart rate acquisition for adherence monitoring using a smart phone platform." *Journal of Alternative and Complementary Medicine* 19(1) (2013): 17–19.

Guimarães, K. C., L. F. Drager, P. R. Genta, et al. "Effects of oropharyngeal exercises on patients with moderate obstructive sleep apnea syndrome." *American Journal of Respiratory and Critical Care Medicine* 179(10) (2009): 962–66.

Hallberg, O., and O. Johansson. "Sleep on the right side—Get cancer on the left?" *Pathophysiology* 17(3) (2010): 157–60.

Halsey, L. G., J. W. Huber, T. Low, et al. "Does consuming breakfast influence activity levels? An experiment into the effect of breakfast consumption on eating habits and energy expenditure." *Public Health Nutrition* 15(2) (2012): 238–45.

Howatson, G., P. G. Bell, J. Tallent, et al. "Effect of tart cherry juice (*Prunus cerasus*) on melatonin levels and enhanced sleep quality." 51(8) (2012): 909–16.

Jones, J. M. "In U.S. 40% get less than recommended amount of sleep." *Gallup* (2013): www.gallup.com/poll/166553/less-recommended-amount-sleep.aspx

Josic, J., A. T. Olsson, J. Wickeberg, et al. "Does green tea affect postprandial glucose, insulin and satiety in healthy subjects: A randomized controlled trial." *Nutrition Journal* 9 (2010): 63.

Lin, H. H., P. S. Tsai, S. C. Fang, and J. F. Liu. "Effect of kiwifruit consumption on sleep quality in adults with sleep problems." *Asia Pacific Journal of Clinical Nutrition* 20(2) (2011): 169–74.

Heaner, M. "Snooze alarm takes its toll on a nation." *New York Times,* October 12, 2004. http://www.nytimes.com/2004/10/12/health/12snoo.html

Roehrs, T. A., S. Randal, E. Harris, et al. "MSLT in primary insomnia: Stability and relation to nocturnal sleep." *Sleep* 34(12) (2011): 1647–52.

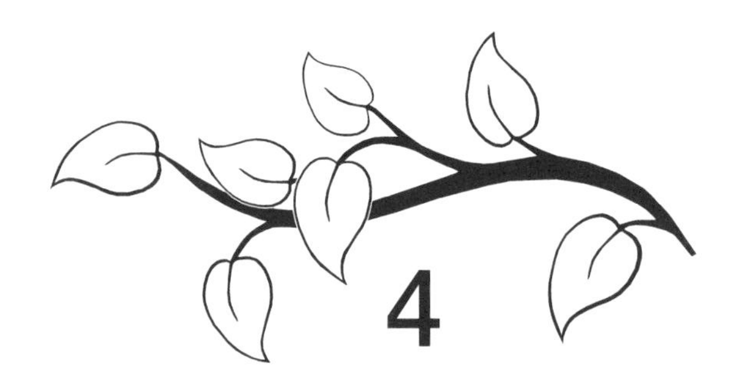

4

COMMONSENSE SOLUTIONS TO EVERYDAY HEALTH PROBLEMS

Sneezing is the poor man's orgasm.

Extract from *L'Os à Moëlle* (The Marrow Bone), Pierre Dac

Medications are useful when taking them is necessary. That seems obvious, and yet it's not always so. In my practice I'm aware of too many illnesses of iatrogenic origin. An iatrogenic illness is an illness that is caused by the secondary effects of a medication—what we commonly call side effects. You could avoid such problems by cavalierly going without prescriptions, but for many conditions this would be ill advised or even dangerous. Unfortunately, though, people have multiple reasons for becoming hooked on medications, including sudden fatigue, recurrent discomfort, or persistent pain. As the months go by, you need to increase the dosage, moving on to more and more aggressive therapies to address the symptoms without ever resolving the origin of what is wrong. There are, however, numerous symptoms in everyday life that can be remedied by simple measures without going to a doctor: constipation, bloating, digestive discomfort, allergies, and breathing difficulties, to name a few. Knowing about these simple solutions makes it possible to cut back on taking medications, reducing dependency and avoiding dangerous or uncomfortable side effects. When it's a question of learning something new that is risk free in order to get rid of a symptom, I am always in favor of the more natural solution.

GASTROENTEROLOGICAL DISORDERS

Gastroenterological disorders (constipation, bloating, hiatal hernia, gastric reflux) are among the most frequent reasons for a visit to the doctor. However, many digestive upsets can be easily avoided by changing how we look after ourselves. To convince you of this, I suggest that you study trees. Trees that grow straight up are quicker to have their tops push up toward the sky. In contrast, the ones that develop bent over cannot expect to live a long life. The difficulty in the case of the human body is that it needs to assume good positions while at the same time being constantly in motion. The ideal is to always place yourself over your center of gravity, whatever body positions are adopted. Movement is essential to life, because, as Einstein said, "Life is like riding a bicycle. To keep your balance, you must keep moving."

The New Posture to Adopt on Toilets

I am going to broach a subject that is sensitive and very private. It has to do with the best positions to assume for defecation. This topic may seem surprising since, as we all know, there's just one position that everyone uses when seated on the throne. However, it may not be the best position. Several teams of researchers in the United States, Israel, and Japan have devoted themselves to this topic, and all the scientific investigations came to the same conclusion: it is better to be in a crouched position rather than seated in order to pass stools. In fact, the seated position is a relatively recent position that developed because of modern toilets, but it is not physiological.

The research has brought to light several new elements. In a seated position the anorectal angle is much more closed compared to the crouched position; such an angle tends to hold back the feces inside the rectum and requires more pushing to pass them, which then often happens incompletely. To illustrate this hypothesis think of a garden hose full of water that is half folded: the water flows through with some difficulty. This is exactly what happens when you are in a seated position. When the subject is in a crouched position, the angle opens, the fold disappears, and the water flows easily.

The doctors who conducted these experiments with volunteers observed that people took three times less time to pass their stools when in a crouched position instead of a seated position. The participants all noted that they hardly needed to push when they were in a crouched position and that the defecation was easy and fast. This detail is very important for those suffering from hemorrhoids since this change of position reduces the pain and the recurrence of crises while reducing pressure in a way that is physiological. In the case of cardiovascular pathologies, the effort to make it happen is limited, which allows the subject to avoid pointless increases in arterial pressure.

At first glance it may seem difficult to put this recommendation into practice since what are sometimes called *Turkish toilets* have almost disappeared in France and are virtually unheard of in the United States. Some people have suggested that you should crouch on the toilet seat, but that might seem a little perilous! There is an in-between solution that consists of placing a little stool in front of the throne to raise your feet when you are seated. Or more simply you can slide your hands under your thighs to raise your legs, straighten up, and automatically you will tilt back. And there you are! Such a position allows you to partially remove the rectal kink that the seated position creates. Participants in the studies noted that they saved an hour a week just because of this position. And moreover, this practice may allow you to avoid using laxatives.

Opting for a better position on the toilet has more advantages than just saving time. It can relieve the suffering of people who have hemorrhoids. Hemorrhoids are dilated vessels in the area of the anus that resemble varicose veins in the legs. They can be very painful and can cause inflammation and bleeding. Reducing the amount of pushing when passing stool will be very beneficial by avoiding an increase in pressure in these blood vessels. Moving to another area, a team of scientists in Taiwan studied the connection in a man between erectile problems and hemorrhoids. The study was conducted on more than six thousand men. They noted that 90 percent of the men suffering from erectile problems in fact had hemorrhoids, and this was even more striking since they were under thirty years of age. The reason seems to be connected to the fact that swelling of certain vessels near the rectum gives rise to an irritation of the nearby nerves involved in an erection. Try out this new position, and judge for yourself how effective it is.

The Dangers of Work Sitting Down

Positions of the body at rest can affect your health. This has been shown by an Australian study conducted with nine hundred patients suffering from colon cancer who were compared to one thousand control-group subjects who were in good health. The scientists put together a database that assembled information on their eating habits and their physical and professional activities. The subjects who worked in a seated position in front of a computer were considered sedentary compared to those whose work required constant movement, such as a nurse or restaurant waiter. The researchers found that subjects who worked in sedentary professions for at least ten years had twice the risk of contracting colon cancer. Among these cancers it is those cancers that are "closest to the seat of the chair" that are the most frequent—especially cancers of the rectum, for which the frequency is 1.5 times as high. It is interesting to realize that this increase in frequency regarding the risk of cancer does not depend on physical activity practiced outside of working hours. This element is fundamental. It means that being in a seated position for eight hours a day, independent of other activities in the day, constitutes a risk factor. A daily sports activity is not enough to offset the days spent seated. And this is not the first study on this subject. Other earlier studies had already suggested that the fact of being seated for too long constituted a risk of colon cancer.

Sedentary Has Got to Go!

When you realize that reducing your time seated to less than three hours a day increases life expectancy, you will likely think twice! I suggest that TV lovers ought to watch their favorite programs while working out on a stationary bike. If you have to spend a lot of time seated, take regular breaks by walking for a few minutes outside your office. If you're at home fold your laundry, scrub your bathtub, clean the windows. In short, always alternate a physical activity with a stationary position. These simple actions will significantly increase your life expectancy in good health. The study that put its finger on this correlation took place in the United States where people often watch TV stretched out on their sofas. The researchers, led by Dr. P. Katzmarzyk of Baton Rouge, Louisiana, insisted on the fact that in a seated position the muscles of the legs and thighs were inactive, therefore contributing to a disruption of the metabolism of sugars and fats in the blood.

In order to understand the link between colonic cancers and a prolonged seated position, the Australian scientists studied the physiological mechanisms that such a position engenders. It seems that being sedentary is a factor that increases glycemia (blood sugar level) and the level of circulating inflammatory molecules. As well, being sedentary is a known factor in being overweight, which is itself an independent cancer risk. Obesity involves an increase in the daily intake of food. It is obvious that when you eat three or four times the quantity necessary for the body, you take in more pesticides and chemical products contained in certain foods. The tolerance standards for such toxic products are based on quantities that I would consider to be normal. Therefore, too high a dose of them can constitute a poison. The human body is not designed to detoxify an excess of food. In this situation the kidneys and the liver, which are natural filters, are overloaded. You need only observe the number of overweight subjects who show a fatty liver in their ultrasound examination. It is exactly the same for ducks and geese: a liver overloaded by such excesses no longer responds to the demand.

Gastroesophageal Reflux

Gastroesophageal reflux (GER) affects a significant number of people. It consists of a movement of acidic liquid back up along the esophagus, sometimes up into the throat; this happens after meals, mainly when the person is in a reclining position. Physiologically, GER is due to poor circulation in the alimentary vessel. When you eat the food descends along your esophagus and then comes to a kind of "muscle-trap" (the cardia). This muscle, which separates your esophagus from your stomach, opens to allow the food to pass and then closes again. In the case of GER, this sphincter isn't sufficiently tonic to close completely, and it allows acidic food particles to move back up from the stomach. If you are suffering from reflux, you clearly need to consult your doctor because a medical treatment can solve the problem. Nevertheless, a few simple hygienic or dietary actions will allow you to prevent and alleviate this very disagreeable problem:

- Don't dive into bed right after eating—raise up the top part of your body using a second pillow.
- Eat small quantities.
- Watch your weight.
- Ban tobacco and alcohol.
- Avoid spicy food, onions, and grease.

Hiatal Hernia

One-third of French people suffer from hiatal hernia, and the condition is similarly cause for concern in the United States. The hiatal hernia is a small part of the stomach that extends up past the diaphragm, causing frequent acid reflux and belching. There are simple and practical methods that can contribute effectively to reducing or eliminating these symptoms without having recourse to the classic medications, which have the inconvenience of having to be taken all year long, not to mention their possible side effects.

First of all you must absolutely avoid drinking or eating burning hot food. This is something I recommend regardless of the hiatal hernia. Drinking something too hot increases the risk of cancer of the esophagus. A study conducted in Jiangsu, China, has clearly shown that drinking tea that is too hot increases the frequency of these cancers. There are other elements at the basis of these cancers, such as tobacco and alcohol, but it turns out that drinks or food at a temperature that is too high is one of the real risks. A healthy drink such as green tea can therefore become harmful to the health if it is drunk burning hot. Here we have a key point in nutrition and healthy eating. It's simply a question of temperature and method of preparation.

While we're speaking about hot drinks, there is another little paradox. Many travelers have noticed that nomads in the desert drink hot tea to cool down. In fact, when the temperature rises, we sweat in order to evaporate water, which causes the body to cool down. When you take a cold drink, you are pushing the body to produce the energy necessary to warm you up. When first drunk there is a sensation of coolness but then you get hot. Conversely, drinking a tea that is slightly warm produces a sensation of coolness that lasts.

In the context of the hiatal hernia, drinking something too hot pushes us to swallow air to cool down the liquid. Swallowing too much air then puts pressure on the stomach, encouraging acid reflux and belching. There are other suggestions to be followed so as to avoid an excessive ingestion of air: don't walk and eat at the same time, don't eat while talking, don't chew gum, and avoid drinking from a straw or directly from the bottle. Of course, you should eat as slowly as possible with your mouth closed.

Bloating

What could be more disagreeable than those moments where, after a meal or at the end of the day, you realize that your stomach is triple its usual size, that it is painful, and that you have the impression you are about to give birth to an elephant! At one time or another, we have all felt such bloating, which generally disappears after a few hours. In medical jargon we call it *functional colonopathy*. The colon whose function is to transport food residue to the "exit" swells up with air, becomes lazy, and functions more slowly, most often provoking constipation. However, numerous doctors will tell you that it is not a "real" disease and that a simple modification of a few nutritional rules is all that is needed to avoid these difficulties. To accomplish that you need to promote a diet that is rich in fiber and you need to drink lots of water. Fibers cannot be assimilated by the body. They move through the digestive apparatus and promote digestion by dragging the remains of food with them. In order to act effectively, they need to swell up, which is why it is important to drink at least 1.5 liters (3.2 pints) of water outside of and during meals. It is equally important to eat slowly and calmly. Everyone has noticed that you don't digest as well after an animated, noisy meal that was eaten hurriedly.

Fiber

Fiber is found in a wide variety of foods:

- Grains (bread, rice, wheat, semolina).
- Legumes (red beans, lentils, chickpeas).
- Vegetables (green beans, spinach, asparagus, celery, fennel, artichokes).
- All fruit.
- Food supplements (carbon, clay) and probiotics are also effective as part of a fiber-rich diet.

ALLERGIES

Allergies today affect a growing segment of the population and are becoming a real public health problem. The Asthma and Allergy Foundation of America estimates that allergies affect approximately fifty million people in the United States. And it is estimated that more than twenty million people in France suffer from allergies, which is a very high number. This figure has doubled in twenty years, and the curve continues to steepen year after year. The effects are multiple, ranging from a bit of itchiness to asthma, from coughing to Quincke's edema, which can be fatal. Why are allergies shooting up? Can we do something to prevent and reduce this phenomenon?

Calves, Cows, and Open Air

Some history books recount how in olden times, in certain well-to-do families, babies were sent at birth to farms where there were wet nurses. They returned much later to their homes spick-and-span, knowing how to talk and walk. Later, in the nineteenth century, the area of Morvan became the breast-feeding capital of France with its famous Morvanian wet nurses. Famous for their breast-feeding talents, these women took in thousands of babies sent from the Paris welfare office. It is estimated that more than fifty thousand children were placed in this way in the Morvan area, which the locals called little Paris. The wet nurses came from modest families that had been further impoverished by the industrial revolution. This is how the writer Jean Genet came to be placed at the age of thirteen in one of these families. The reputation of these wet nurses was such that Napoléon I, on the advice of his doctor, engaged a Morvanian wet nurse to breast-feed his son Napoléon II, King of Rome. Later the president of France, Félix Faure, did the same. Once having returned to the countryside, the wet nurses came back with enough money to buy a house, which the local inhabitants called milk houses. Although the long-past practice of sending children to the farm could be criticized from the perspective of emotional relationships, perhaps without knowing it these people discovered the first effective method of preventing allergies.

A team of German researchers in fact has recently made a fascinating discovery. They compared several thousand children living on farms with a group of children living in the city. These are two completely different environments. In the first case life on a farm implies daily contact with many animals such as cows, pigs, and chickens. In the second case it is a much more sterile world. The result of these studies clearly showed that children who grew up on a farm developed considerably fewer allergies than children from cities, with a 51 percent reduction in the risk of asthma and 76 percent in the risk of allergies. It is possible that it was the early contact with all the microbes of the farm that made the difference. In fact, in the rural environment there is a great diversity of fungi, bacteria, and all kinds of microorganisms that would have a beneficial immunizing effect right from the beginnings of life. It seems that the preventive effect of this contact with farm animals in childhood continues into adulthood.

The Dog—Man's Best Friend

In the same vein we need to cite recent studies having to do with the connections between the presence of a dog in the home and childhood asthma. It seems that the microbes naturally present with a dog could play a role in fighting the respiratory syncytial virus that is connected to asthmatic crises in children. The scientific studies used mice that had been exposed to dust from houses where dogs lived. It seems that the mice were then protected from this virus. This research is based on the empirical finding that children who live in contact with dogs developed less asthma. In fact, early contact with dogs in childhood stimulates immune system defenses in a positive way.

Kissing and Allergies

An allergen can be transmitted with a kiss. If you are allergic to peanuts and your partner has just eaten some, a kiss can set off a severe allergic reaction because of particles of this food that could be transmitted in an exchange of saliva. This can range from simple itchiness to the fearsome Quincke's edema. It's the ideal scenario for a detective novel called *The Kiss That Kills*. But all is not lost—far from it! Let's not forget the astonishing research of Dr. Kimata in Japan, who showed that prolonged kissing in couples led to a decrease in allergies. To accomplish this he studied twenty-four couples where one of each couple was suffering from moderate eczema. He asked them to kiss freely as often as possible for thirty minutes. Just before beginning and right after the thirty minutes, he drew blood samples to test for biological constants (IgE) that are associated with allergies. The results showed a decrease in the biological blood agent for the allergy being studied and a decrease in eczema in those so affected.

LITERATURE

Almqvist, C., F. Garden, A. S. Kemp, et al. "Effects of early cat or dog ownership on sensitisation and asthma in a high-risk cohort without disease-related modification of exposure." *Paediatric and Perinatal Epidemiology* 24(2) (2010): 171–78.

Billhult, A., C. Lindholm, R. Gunnarsson, and E. Stener-Vicorin. "The effect of massage on cellular immunity, endocrine and psychological factors in women with breast cancer—a randomized controlled clinical trial." *Autonomic Neuroscience* 140(1–2) (2008): 88–95.

Boyle, T., L. Fritschi, J. Heyworth, and F. Bull. "Long-term sedentary work and the risk of subsite-specific colorectal cancer." *American Journal of Epidemiology* 173(10) (2011): 1183–91.

Cady, S. H., and G. E. Jones. "Massage therapy as a workplace intervention for reduction of stress." *Perceptual and Motor Skills* 84(1) (1997): 157–58.

Clark, C. E., R. S. Taylor, A. C. Shore, and J. L. Campbell. "The difference in blood pressure readings between arms and survival: Primary care cohort study." *BMJ: British Medical Journal* 344 (2012): e1327.

Clark, C. E., R. S. Taylor, A. C. Shore. et al. "Association of a difference in systolic blood pressure between arms with vascular disease and mortality: A systematic review and meta-analysis." *Lancet* 379(9819) (2012): 905–14.

Cooper, R., D. Kuh, R. Hardy, et al. "Objectively measured physical capability levels and mortality: Systematic review and meta-analysis." *BMJ: British Medical Journal* 341 (2010): c4467.

Ever-Hadani, P., D. S. Seidman, O. Manor, and S. Harlap. "Breast feeding in Israel: Maternal factors associated with choice and duration." *Journal of Epidemiology and Community Health* 48(3) (1994): 281–85.

Fugimura, K. E., T. Demoor, M. Rauch, et al. "House dust exposure mediates gut microbiome *Lactobacillus* enrichment and airway immune defense against allergens and virus infection." *Proceedings of the National Academy of Sciences* 111(2) (2014): 805–10.

Green, J., B. J. Cairns, D. Casabonne, et al. "Height and cancer incidence in the Million Women Study: Prospective cohort, and meta-analysis of prospective studies of height and total cancer risk." *Lancet Oncology* 12(8) (2011): 785–94.

Grewen. K. M., S. S. Girdler, J. Amico, and K. C. Light. "Effects of partner support on resting oxytocin, cortisol, neuropinephrine, and blood pressure before and after warm partner contact." *Psychosomatic Medicine* 67(4) (2005) 531–38.

Katzmarzyk, P. T., T. S. Church, C. L. Craig, and C. Bouchard. "Sitting time and mortality from all causes, cardiovascular disease, and cancer." *Medicine and Science in Sports and Exercise* 41(5) (2009): 998–1005.

Keller, J. J., and H. C. Lin. "Haemorrhoids are associated with erectile dysfunction: A population-based study." *International Journal of Andrology* 35(6) (2012): 867–72.

Kimata, H. "Kissing selectively decreases allergen-specific IgE production in atopic patients." *Journal of Psychosomatic Research* 60(5) (2006): 545–47.

Lerro, C. C., K. A. McGlynn, and M. B. Cook. "A systematic review and meta-analysis of the relationship between body size and testicular cancer." *British Journal of Cancer* 103(9) (2010): 1467–74.

Lin, H. H., P. S. Tsai, S. C. Fang, and J. F. Liu. "Effect of kiwifruit consumption on sleep quality in adults with sleep problems." *Asia Pacific Journal of Clinical Nutrition* 20(2) (2011): 169–74.

Löberbauer-Purer, E., N. L. Meyer, S. Ring-Dimitriou, et al. "Can alternating lower body negative and positive pressure during exercise alter regional body fat distribution or skin appearance?" *European Journal of Applied Physiology* 112(5) (2012): 1861–71.

Maloney, J. M., M. D. Chapman, and S. H. Sicherer. "Peanut allergen exposure through saliva: Assessment and interventions to reduce exposure." *Journal of Allergy and Clinical Immunology* 118(3) (2006): 719–24.

Muller, D. C., G. G. Giles, J. T. Manning, et al. "Second to fourth digit ratio (2D: 4D) and prostate cancer risk in the Melbourne Collaborative Cohort Study." *British Journal of Cancer* 105(3) (2011): 438–40.

Rao, S. S., R. Kavlock, and S. Rao. "Influence of body position and stool characteristics on defecation in humans." *American Journal of Gastroenterology* 101(12) (2006): 2790–96.

Sikirov, D. "Comparison of straining during defecation in three positions: Results and implications for human health." *Digestive Diseases and Sciences* 48(7) (2003): 1201–5.

Von Ehrenstein, O. S., E. Von Mutius, S. Illi, et al. "Reduced risk of asthma and hayfever among children of farmers." *Clinical and Experimental Allergy* 30(2) (2000): 187–93.

Waser, M., E. von Mutius, J. Riedler, et al. "Exposition aux animaux domestiques et leur association avec le rhume des foins, l'asthme et la sensibilisation atopique chez des enfants en milieu rural." *Allergy* 60(2) (2005): 177–84; article in French.

Wiesner, J., and A. Vilcinskas. "Antimicrobial peptides: The ancient arm of the human immune system." *Virulence* 1(5) (2010): 440–64.

Wu, M., A. M. Liu, E. Kampman, et al. "Green tea drinking, high tea temperature and esophageal cancer in high- and low-risk areas of Jiangsu Province, China: A population-based case-control study." *International Journal of Cancer* 124(8) (2009): 1907–13.

Zhao, K. Q., A. T. Cowan, R. J. Lee, et al. "Molecular modulation of airway epithelial ciliary response to sneezing." *FASEB Journal* 26(8) (2012): 3178–87.

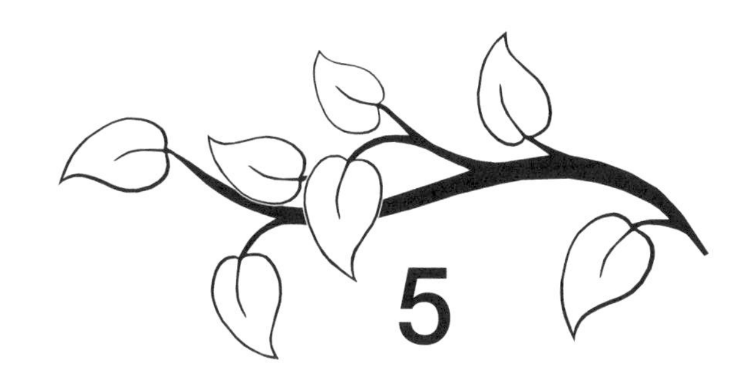

5

THE STRUGGLE AGAINST INFECTIOUS DISEASES AND HOW TO PROTECT YOUR CHILDREN

Don't underestimate small adversaries: you can see a lion but not a virus.

Anonymous

An infection—here we have a common term that we use every day. An infection is the invasion of a living organism by microbes that can be of diverse origin, including virus, bacteria, and fungus. Such an invasion is capable of leading to illness, which is why their agents are pathogens. An infection can be exogenous (the environment bringing in germs), endogenous (the individual produces the germs), nosocomial (the patient develops the infection following a hospital stay), or finally, opportunistic (the infection develops in a healthy individual, but does not lead to illness in so far as the organism defends itself well). It is important to remember that an infection most often develops in an individual whose immune system has been weakened. To use a warrior metaphor, if you are attacked by the enemy and your castle is not well protected, you run the risk of very quickly being invaded! This chapter, like earlier chapters, does not intend to minimize the seriousness of infectious disease, but rather to provide you with lots of preventive measures so that you can reinforce your organism. A well-maintained body is naturally more able to resist disease.

DAILY HYGIENE: NEITHER TOO MUCH NOR NOT ENOUGH

Could it be that excessive hygiene and antibiotics in early childhood are the reason for the rise in the occurrence of allergies we previously discussed? Is it possible that the ultrasterile world in which we are living contributes to autoimmune, inflammatory, and infectious diseases?

Habits We Don't Always Think About

Good hygiene is clearly essential in avoiding the pointless development of many infections all year long. It is important therefore to acquire good daily habits. In an earlier book* I reminded people of the importance of ground rules that are unfortunately often forgotten because hygiene is no longer, or rarely, taught in school, nor is it taught in medical school or even by mothers to their children. But hygiene really works! Let's mention here a few examples:

- The simple fact of washing your hands before having a meal or after leaving the toilet reduces respiratory or digestive infections by 20 percent.
- Closing the toilet cover before flushing avoids the aerosol effect by means of which germs can make their way into the lungs.

*Frédéric Saldmann, *Wash Your Hands: Dirty Truth About Germs, Viruses, and Epidemics . . . and the Simple Ways to Protect Yourself in a Dangerous World* (New York: Weinstein Books, 2008).

- Changing your pillow regularly is important because at the end of two years, 10 percent of its weight is due to household dust mites or their feces.
- Washing your refrigerator twice a month is basic because of the risk of microbial growths—such as the fearsome *Listeria*—which develop precisely in such cold, damp atmospheres at 40 degrees Fahrenheit.
- Freezing fish that you want to eat raw eliminates anisakis, a parasite that may be the cause of intestinal punctures; doing the same with steak that you want to eat tartare avoids contracting tapeworm, which happens to 100,000 individuals in France every year.
- You need to know that certain kinds of food don't keep—such as all raw meat or fish and also fresh mayonnaise.
- Remember that what you use to clean up with can end up being a fearsome carrier of filth. The sponge can become a haven for microbes if you don't rinse it with bleach regularly before letting it dry. Dishcloths need to be washed as often as possible at 140 degrees Fahrenheit and should never be reused if they are wet.
- You should never share your bath towel with the whole family; passing the bath towel around means passing microbes around. Also, be careful to let your towel dry before using it. If it is still wet, don't hesitate to put it in the laundry basket. In fact, a wet towel is a perfect culture environment for microbe development. In twenty-four hours they have plenty of time to reproduce. The result is that once your cleanup time is over, you will have spread colonies of microbes over yourself that then develop with a clear preference for folds of skin, promoting rashes and infections. Rubber gloves should only be used once in the bathroom and then washed. Otherwise, on the second usage they will simply spread filth over your body.

Handwashing That Chases Away Bad Feelings

Handwashing can take on a psychological and symbolic dimension. It's an activity that allows you to distance yourself from bad feelings, doubts, and negative thoughts. This is what Dr. Spike Lee, while studying at the University of Michigan, became aware of in speaking to people who had washed their hands. I think that it is still an effective hygienic thing to do and a precaution against the possible transmission to others. If you can eliminate microbes and negative thoughts at the same time, that's one more reason to remember this healthy daily habit!

- I recommend washing your sheets at least once a week. Remember also to regularly change your toothbrush, especially after flu or a sore throat so as to avoid reinfection and dragging out infections that never seem to end. To economize on toothbrushes I advise you to quite simply put them in the dishwasher with the usual detergent. A scientific study has shown that this method completely eliminates all microbes that were present. After all, you wash your plate every day, why not wash your toothbrush too?
- For plates that are not going straight into the dishwasher, rinse them with a little bleach in order to avoid creating a breeding ground that's just waiting to happen in your kitchen.
- Also consider using a sponge and bleach to properly maintain the rubber sealing strips in your dishwasher, which are often contaminated with mold.
- Obviously, you ought to do a regular cleanup on objects of daily use such as television remotes, bedside-table light switches, cell phones, glasses, and the back of your watch. When you realize that 92 percent of portable phones are covered in microbes, of which 16 percent are fecal bacteria, it is a strong motivation to clean them and, in any case, to also avoid loaning them and exchanging microbes in so doing—and perhaps at the same time you will reduce your phone bill.

Washing Your Body in the Right Direction

When washing your body you should always start from the top down. The reason is simple. It's better to begin with the parts that are cleaner and finish with the dirtier ones, such as the feet, so that you avoid moving germs on the soap from the feet and buttocks toward the face. Doing things in this order also gives a more logical sense to the flow of water. Speaking about more intimate matters, many vaginal infections could be avoided by not wiping the buttocks back and forth from the anus toward the vagina, but only from the vagina toward the back in order to avoid the migration of microbes from the sides of the anus toward the vagina. That all seems logical, however not everyone thinks about it.

Turn Your Cup Around

If you find yourself in a café with questionable hygiene and you notice that the waiter has made a very perfunctory washing of the cups by holding them upside down for one second over a small water jet, you would be disgusted and well you should be. There are diseases that can be transmitted by simple contact. Drinking right after someone who has contracted labial herpes or gastroenteritis is not recommended. If in doubt one simple move can lower the risk of transmission: instead of picking up the cup with the handle on the right, turn it and put the handle on the left. Since most people use their cup with the handle on the right, you'll be able to drink your coffee from the side least used by others.

DOES TOO MUCH HYGIENE KILL HYGIENE?

Finding the Right Balance

It is clear that progress in cleanliness has contributed in a spectacular way to reducing the frequency of infection and extending life expectancy. However, sometimes, there can be too much of a good thing. Too much hygiene kills hygiene. The hard thing is to find the perfect balance between necessary and basic ground rules and a hygiene that is pathological. I will begin with a very telling example: antiseptic products or soap should never be used to clean the vagina! These products will literally destroy the internal organic balance of the flora and lead to the opposite of the desired result—repeated vaginal infections for example. You need to keep in mind that the vagina is like a self-cleaning oven in that it does not need special products for its intimate maintenance. Along the same lines too many antibiotics, when they are not necessary, can lead to a variety of resistant bacterial strains and break the balance of the intestinal flora. The concept of microbial ecology is fundamental. The human body carries millions of germs that form a stable equilibrium. We need to think about doing as much as we can to maintain this fragile balance.

Numerous investigations on the strange connections between certain microbes and asthma raise certain questions. The example of a gastric ulcer is very much to the point. When I was a medical student, gastric ulcers were considered to be a psychosomatic disease due to too much stress. Fearsome complications could result from them such as gastric perforation with hemorrhaging and peritonitis. A significant number of patients underwent surgical interventions involving an ablation of the stomach that made the rest of their lives very painful, requiring them to eat very small quantities at each meal. But there was a treatment that was unknown and could have been prescribed. Many years later a researcher discovered that gastric ulcers were very simply linked to a bacteria: *Helicobacter pylori.* Antibiotic treatment can get rid of it. But now recent scientific studies have produced an embarrassing fact—they make clear that the presence of *Helicobacter pylori* reduces the frequency of asthma in patients with asthmatic conditions.

Through the web of results from these studies, we can glimpse a gamut of difficulties in the relationships among hygiene, the immune system, and allergies. The organism has to "grow teeth" as it progressively enters into contact with various microbes so that it can build a solid immunity, and at the same time it is essential to protect the organism from infectious agents that are too dangerous. The border between managing microbes or toxins and good health is not so simple. The botulinum toxin used to get rid of wrinkles or to reduce certain spasms is also a poison that can kill.

The Benefits of Sneezing

Someone who has just sneezed or coughed on his own hands has just covered them with viruses. Shaking hands with others right afterward is an opportunity to contaminate the whole gathering, all within a context of irreproachable civility. The right reflex is to sneeze or cough against one's sleeve or to use a single-use handkerchief or a tissue. In practical terms sneezing can be a means of propagating the virus from someone with a cold, and moreover this takes place at 200 kilometers an hour (125 miles per hour). It's a fast way of spreading viral disease.

When a person sneezes it is common for those around to interpret this as a negative phenomenon. *Gesundheit* or *bless you* are the common currency of exchange. In fact, in the light of new scientific investigation, it seems that sneezing is very good for your health. Sneezing allows you to clear microbes that accumulate in the nasal passages. The violent exhalation of air is like the stroke of a whip for the nasal mucus that is in charge of getting rid of bacteria, viruses, and the residues of urban pollution. It is like a ventilation and air purification system being put in place. So don't hesitate to use this perfectly healthy system for expelling your miasmas into a handkerchief followed by a hand wash afterward.

Sneezing through the Ages and in Different Cultures

In the Middle Ages many people thought that when you sneezed, a devil could enter your mouth, which gave rise to using your hand as a kind of protection. This custom has persisted through the ages. Depending on the culture sneezing can take on numerous meanings: for the Japanese, if you sneeze once, it means someone is speaking well of you; if twice, someone is speaking ill of you; if three times, it's a lover speaking about you; if more than that, you have a cold.

VACCINATING KISSES

The Secret of Saliva

The saliva that is exchanged in a kiss carries special properties that have been recently discovered. It contains a protein, SLPI. This component of saliva has powerful biological effects that combat microbes, mycoses, and certain viruses. These facts help us understand why the transmission of the AIDS virus by mouth is extremely rare. In addition, this protein helps in healing tissues and has anti-inflammatory effects. A team of researchers at the National Institutes of Health in Bethesda, Maryland, applied this fabulous protein to the skin of mice that had wounds. Forty-eight hours later the mice were healed. Perhaps here we have the explanation of animals who lick their wounds and of children who ask their parents to kiss their little wounds to make them better. Kisses are also going to add a bonus of saliva to the two partners, promoting the neutralization of acids, and the struggle against dental plaque and cavities by clearing away residual food particles. The influx of saliva boosts the antibacterial protein, which is excellent for the teeth.

Transitory Monogamy Rewarded

Kissing at the beginning of a love relationship involving an exchange of saliva between lovers helps the future mother avoid one day transmitting a terrible viral disease to her baby. Through the kisses she immunizes herself against cytomegaloviruses. This virus is caught when you kiss. Most of the time the virus passes unnoticed and is neutralized spontaneously and without consequence. At the most the person feels a little tired, with a few aches and a light fever that is put down to a passing flu. However, thanks to this viral contact, the woman immunizes herself against cytomegaloviruses for life. It is important to acquire a good protection since this disease, benign in an adult, is terrible for the fetus with the possibility of severe intellectual disability, deafness, and liver attacks. The optimal immunity occurs about six months after the first kiss, but there is one small downside. There are different strains of this virus, which means that the woman will be protected only against a single strain, the one that her initial partner transmitted to her. In short, each man carries a specific strain of the virus. This would suggest that monogamy in the six months preceding conception of a baby is a good thing. However, note that a young woman who has engaged in numerous kisses with multiple partners will be immunized against numerous strains of this virus. This medical knowledge illustrates the power of kisses as immunity boosters through exchange of saliva between partners.

PROTECTING ONE'S CHILDREN

Breast-feeding: Beneficial for Children and for Mothers

Mothers or future moms who are reading this, please realize that this paragraph is not intended to make you feel guilty. Breast-feeding is a choice, and for medical reasons or personal reasons, you are totally free to not breast-feed your child. My reason for speaking about breast-feeding here is that it is extremely beneficial for health and not only the health of the child. We generally think of all the advantages of breast-feeding for the newborn, but we forget the strong points for the mom. It is surprising to realize to what an extent breast-feeding is relevant to disease prevention and health. It reduces the risk of ovarian, uterine, and breast cancer. It also protects against osteoporosis. A Norwegian team studied a group of five thousand women aged fifty to ninety-four for a period of fifteen years. They discovered that the women who had breast-fed had two times less risk of fractures of the head of the femur than women who had not breast-fed. They also found that breast-feeding leads to a reduction in the need for insulin in diabetic mothers. In addition, since it has an action of blocking ovulation, it is clear that it contributes to a better conservation of the precious stock of oocytes, and perhaps therefore a shift in the age of menopause (see text box on page 68). The duration of lactation varies a lot between countries and cultures. In France women breast-feed for ten weeks on the average; the average duration of breast-feeding in the United States is three months, according to The National Association for Child Development. In Africa this period extends up to two years and, with the Inuit, up to seven years. So, given the numerous positive effects, if it is possible, why not prolong the breast-feeding period? Can breast-feeding take place outside of pregnancy? And what if breast-feeding became a factor in disease prevention and health in its own right? It is perfectly possible to breast-feed without having been pregnant, and for example, this could interest women who adopt or who have their baby carried to term by another woman because of infertility. It is important to know that the two hormones that release breast milk, prolactin and oxytocin, can be activated outside of pregnancy. It is the pituitary gland located in the brain that controls their production and not the ovaries as one might think. It is therefore a simple question of mechanical stimulation of the breast that releases the flow of milk. The work of stimulating the breast, which the nursing baby does instinctively, can be produced mechanically outside of pregnancy. In practice, to achieve this result you need to mechanically make about twelve stimulations a day, something that can be done with a breast pump.

Another point is that the milk from a woman who is breast-feeding a baby of eighteen months is just as rich as the milk from a woman who is nursing an infant of three months. Certain studies tend to show that it might even be a little richer. A group of Israeli researchers compared the milk of women who were nursing from two to six months with the milk of women who nursed for thirty-nine months. For the first group the average fat content of the milk was 7 percent compared to 11 percent for the second group. A liter of milk from the women in group one corresponded to 740 calories compared to 880 calories for group two. For the mother the output of energy required to produce a liter of milk also varied from 740 calories to 880 calories, which is a lot. Breast-feeding, which benefits the child by reinforcing immunity, also has an impact on future health. Scientific studies have shown that allergies such as hay fever, for example, occurred less frequently in children who had been breast-fed for more than six months. The risk of allergies decreased by 29 percent with a breast-feeding period between six and twelve months and by 64 percent with breast-feeding that lasted more than a year. The mother also benefits from a prolongation of breast-feeding by a reduction in the risk of developing type 2 diabetes. Scientific studies have shown that women who breast-fed for at least a year had a 15 percent reduction in the risk of diabetes compared to those who had never breast-fed. Moreover, each additional year of breast-feeding further reduced the risk by 15 percent. In other words, after two years of breast-feeding, the risk of developing diabetes in the remainder of her life is reduced by 30 percent, which is considerable when you know the frequency of this affliction in later years. It seems then that maternal breast-feeding engages a beneficial cycle as much for the mother as for the child. In addition, the loss of weight will be faster after the first six months following childbirth. It is important however to be vigilant and monitor a woman who breast-feeds over a long period to make sure that she does not develop any deficiencies. If that happens the doctor will check the food intake and, if need be, can prescribe appropriate food supplements.

Every year new studies are published that bring out new reasons for breast-feeding, especially over the long term. Seeing breast-feeding as an approach to disease prevention and health for the mother as well as for the child is a new medical dimension.

Breast-feeding stimulated outside of pregnancy opens another avenue of research. If we carry the reasoning forward, what would be the result of daily lactation for a year using a breast pump for a woman outside the maternal context? There is a deep taboo here, but it merits thinking about. What would the impact be on weight, on the risk of diabetes, and on the frequency of gynecological cancer?

Delaying Menopause

In the course of a woman's life, the number of oocytes (female sexual cells that support reproduction) decreases every year, and it is clear that economizing them makes good sense. The average age of menopause is fifty, but there are significant variations from one woman to the next ranging from forty-five to fifty-five years of age. Menopause corresponds to the end of the supply of ovarian oocytes. Numerous factors come into play to explain the span of up to ten years in the onset of menopause. It is clear that we need to do all we can to delay this onset for as long as possible because menopause is accompanied by many negative elements such as an increase in cardiovascular risk, the risk of osteoporosis, and skin problems corresponding overall to a speeding up of aging. There are ethnic factors—such as the fact that Japanese women enjoy a later menopause. Other nongenetic data elements that we can do something about also enter into the picture. In an earlier book* I highlighted the link between cholesterol levels, blood pressure, smoking, and the age when menopause begins. By modifying certain parameters it is possible to shift this age to up to seven years later. The reason is simple: the vessels that irrigate the ovaries are tiny and sensitive to changes that make them less efficient in tissue irrigation. Such alterations precipitate a lowering of the ovarian supply.

*Frédéric Saldmann, *La Vie et le Temps* [Life and Time], (Paris: Flammarion, 2011).

Catching Toxoplasmosis

Toxoplasmosis is a disease that is one of the zoonoses. Zoonoses are diseases that are transmitted to humans by animals. In the case of toxoplasmosis, the animals concerned are most importantly cats (which by the way are often contaminated by eating mice), but also sheep (two-thirds of them), pigs (one-quarter of them), and cattle in fewer numbers. It is possible to find out if a cat is carrying this disease by giving it laboratory tests, which is important since a positive result is generally not accompanied by any specific symptoms. Contamination from the animal to a person takes place either by living in contact with cats or by eating raw meat or meat that is not cooked enough. In adults the disease is not serious. It resembles an ordinary flu with very little temperature, fleeting muscular aches, fatigue, and some swollen glands. Without any treatment everything spontaneously returns to normal in a week. In some cases the subject has no symptoms and the illness goes by unnoticed. The only risk with this disease is for pregnant women. In fact, if an expectant mother catches toxoplasmosis during her pregnancy, she endangers her fetus who can fall victim to a congenital toxoplasmosis—the terrible neurological or ocular complications of which in extreme cases can lead to blindness. When an expectant mother shows a negative blood test at the beginning of pregnancy, she should have regular blood tests and follow a number of recommendations:

- Stay away from cats.
- Avoid lamb.
- Have all meat well done.
- Carefully wash all fruit and raw food, including prepared salads.
- Avoid handling earth or doing gardening.

When a woman knows from a simple blood test that she has never had toxoplasmosis, it is recommended, during the time she is using contraception and when she is certain she is not pregnant, that she expose herself to this disease by playing with cats or by eating leg of lamb that is nicely pink for example. By catching this benign illness, she may be able to protect her baby in this way when she comes to embark on pregnancy. Unfortunately, most times, the first blood test for toxoplasmosis takes place at the beginning of pregnancy, and after that you have to take all possible measures to avoid this disease.

ORGANS THAT ARE NOT AS USELESS AS ALL THAT

Tonsils and Appendix

It's true . . . you can live without them. I've often heard this said after the removal of an appendix or tonsils. In certain cases the only choice is to surgically remove these organs since, infected, they risk putting the life in danger. However, nowadays things have changed. Doctors carefully weight the pros and cons before whisking the patient to the operating room. In the case of appendicitis, progress in imaging and ultrasound scanning now means that pointless operations can be avoided. And with tonsils medical treatment is always the first choice before considering an operation that in former times, was routine at the slightest sore throat.

The difference is that we know today that these organs play an active role in the body's struggle against infection. Tonsils are active in immune-system defenses. Situated at the entry point of the passageways for air and for food, they are a first-line defense in combating microbes. If they are removed antigen cells can of course continue to be produced in other organs such as glands and marrow.

The number of appendicitis operations in France has gone from 300,000 to 83,000 in twenty years. Two factors are involved in explaining these figures: more precise diagnostic methods and also a better understanding of the functions of this organ, which no longer seems like a useless add-on. Some researchers have shown that it could play a role as a reservoir of good bacteria that would be capable of recolonizing the intestine after serious diarrhea as well as contributing to the production of antigen cells to protect against infections. Recently Dr. Rodney Mason's team in the United States has been experimenting with the use of antibiotics for the treatment of appendicitis, which opens a new avenue of research in the control of this malady.

The Subtle Power of Body Hair

In our present-day society, body hair has fallen out of favor. Men are wearing beards or moustaches less and less, and women pile on depilatory creams, permanent or semipermanent hair removal, laser, wax—everything is marshaled in the struggle against body hair. Scientific discoveries, however, are teaching us uses of body hair unknown up until now. The study that was conducted in fact showed that body hair contributed to the combat against parasites such as bugs. The hair slows down their movement on the skin and makes it easier to notice their intrusion than on hairless skin, allowing the victim to eliminate them with the back of the hand. It's perhaps the reason why humans are the only species of primates victimized by lice.

THE LOOK THAT PROTECTS

Many people fear being in contact with sick people. Fear of disease and of being contaminated keeps people away. As a doctor I am often asked, "How is it that you doctors who are constantly in contact with sick people don't catch all those microbes?" Just being properly vaccinated against flu, hepatitis, and other illnesses does not explain everything. A recent study conducted by a brilliant team of Canadian researchers at the University of British Columbia overturns the popular thinking about this.

Looking at Sick People Boosts the Immune System

The researchers found that having subjects look for ten minutes at unpleasant photos of sick people increased the activation of the subjects' immune-system defenses. The snapshots showed people suffering from severe infectious diseases with rumbling coughs, thick discharges from the nose, festering boils, sores, and all kinds of really overt infectious manifestations. The scientists then took blood samples from the subjects and exposed the blood in the samples to infectious agents. The analyses showed that the subjects who had looked at the photos had produced, in their white blood cells, a one-quarter increase in their cytokines, which are the elements that intercede at the level of the quality of the immune-system response.

In practical terms their immune system was better prepared to respond to infectious agents. Other studies have been conducted based on the hypothesis that what boosted the immune system was in fact the stimulation itself regardless of the agent employed. The researchers presented threatening photos of armed men. The results showed no meaningful difference in level of immunity from the previous tests. In any case this surprising study could perhaps change the attitude of those who tend to flee from sick people as though from the plague.

LITERATURE

Amedei, A., G. Codolo, G. Del Prete, et al. "The effect of *Helicobacter pylori* on asthma and allergy." *Journal of Asthma and Allergy* 3 (2010): 139–47.

Arnold, I. C., N. Dehzad, S. Reuter, et al. "*Helicobacter pylori* infection prevents allergic asthma in mouse models through the induction of regulatory T cells." *Journal of Clinical Investigation* 121(8) (2011): 3088–93.

Ashcroft, G. S., K. Lei, W. Jin, et al. "Secretory leukocyte protease inhibitor mediates non-redundant functions necessary for normal wound healing." *Nature Medicine* 6 (2000): 1147–53.

Au, G. G., L. G. Beagley, E. S. Haley, et al. "Oncolysis of malignant human melanoma tumors by Coxsackieviruses A13, A15 and A18." *Virology Journal* 8(22) (2011): doi: 10.1186/1743-422X-8-22.

Bjørnerem, A., L. A. Ahmed, L. Jørgensen, et al. "Breast-feeding protects against hip fracture in postmenopausal women: The Tromsø study." *Journal of Bone and Mineral Research* 26(12) (2011): 2843–50.

Dean, I., and M. T. Siva Jethy. "Human fine body hair enhances ectoparasite detection." *Biology Letters* 8 (2012): 358–61.

D'Elios, M. M., and M. de Bernard. "To treat or not to treat *Helicobacter pylori* to benefit asthma patients." *Expert Review of Respiratory Medicine* 4(2) (2010): 147–50.

D'Elios, M. M., G. Codolo, A. Amadei. et al. "*Helicobacter pylori*, asthma and allergy." *FEMS Immunology and Medical Microbiology* 56(1) (2009): 1–8.

Ege, M. J., M. Mayer, A. C. Normand, et al. "Exposure to environmental microorganisms and childhood asthma." *New England Journal of Medicine* 364(8) (2011): 701–9.

Ever-Hadani, P., D. S. Seidman, O. Manor, and S. Harlap. "Breast feeding in Israel: Maternal factors associated with choice and duration." *Journal of Epidemiology and Community Health* 48(3) (1994): 281–85.

Freudenheim, J. L., J. R. Marshall, J. E. Vena, et al. "Lactation history and breast cancer risk." *American Journal of Epidemiology* 146(11) (1997): 932–38.

Hendrie, C. A., and G. Brewer. "Kissing as an evolutionary adaptation to protect against human cytomegalovirus-like teratogenesis." *Medical Hypotheses* 74(2) (2010): 222–24.

Kao, L. S., D. Boone, R. J. Mason, et al. "Antibiotics vs appendectomy for uncomplicated acute appendicitis." *Journal of the American College of Surgeons* 216(3) (2013): 501–5.

Lee, S. W., and N. Schwarz. "Dirty hands and dirty mouths: Embodiment of the moral-purity metaphor is specific to the motor modality involved in moral transgression." *Psychological Science* 21(10) (2010): 1423–25.

Presl, J. "Pregnancy and breast feeding decreases the risk of ovarian carcinoma." *Ceskoslovenská Gynekologie* 46(7) (1981): 541–44; article in Czech.

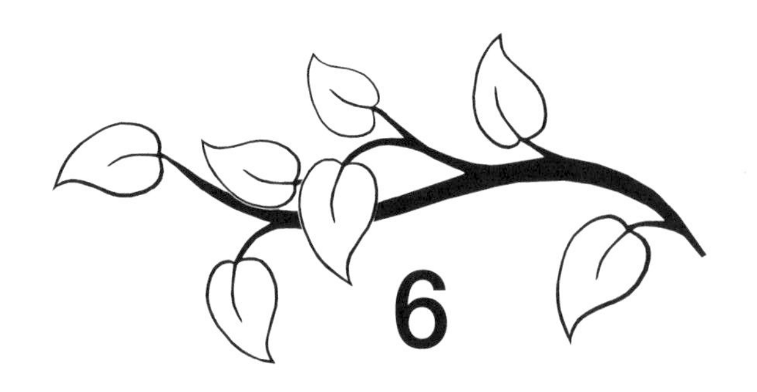

6

PRESSURE POINT THERAPIES FOR EMERGENCIES AND EVERYDAY CARE

True freedom is to have ascendency over all aspects of oneself.

Michel de Montaigne

For many, many symptoms there are simple, manual solutions for treating and healing without having recourse to chemical molecules. One need only activate precise anatomical points on the body to stimulate physiological reactions. The idea of manual treatment came to me through the study of cardiology. Even in such a rigorous discipline, it does happen that we treat patients with our bare hands, such as cardiac massage (CPR) for example. It's one of the most beautiful procedures in cardiology. Just imagine that by exerting regular pressure at one spot on the chest, you can revive someone who was dead a few moments before. You can also treat cardiac illnesses with the fingers. The first time I saw this was when I was a medical student. The subject was a young man of sixteen with AVNRT, a type of tachycardia (fast rhythm) of the heart. AVNRT is characterized by sharp accelerations of the heart happening intermittently. The heart, which normally beats between 70 and

80 times per minute, can peak at up to 250 times a minute. The young man was pale, covered in sweat, and felt like he was on his way out. I watched the on-duty intensive care physician use his fingers to massage a precise point on the neck, and within a few seconds, as if he had tripped a switch, a release took place. In one beat the heart suddenly returned to its normal rhythm. The boy's skin regained its usual color. He no longer felt anything wrong. By exerting pressure on an anatomical point, a physiological reaction had been produced. I discovered that, beyond cardiology, there were many points on the human body that, when activated properly, bring about healing. Whenever possible learn how to fix things yourself without having recourse to a doctor or druggist.

MANAGING EMERGENCY SITUATIONS

Cardiac Arrest and Pathologies of the Heart

In France 50.000 people die every year from cardiac arrest. That number has been reported as 325,000 in the United States. I deeply regret that cardiac massage (CPR) is not better known; indeed, fewer than 20 percent of those who happen to witness cardiac arrest know how to perform it. I believe in the principle that it's better to have an amateur cardiac massage than not to have a cardiac massage at all. Doing nothing means giving the victim no chance of survival. If you happen to witness this one day, here are the basics of what you need to do:

- Verify that the patient is unconscious.
- Call emergency (911 in the USA and Canada).
- With the victim lying flat on a firm surface, place your hands one over the other right in the middle of the chest, keeping your arms locked straight.
- Press down about one hundred times a minute using the whole weight of your body to depress the chest cavity a few inches.
- Completely let go after each compression and continue working until help arrives.

Don't hesitate to keep doing the cardiac massage as long as possible. In 1998, following a cardiac arrest in the operating room, Jean-Pierre Chevènement, a government minister, had the benefit of a cardiac massage that lasted fifty-seven minutes. The heart began beating again after almost an hour of massage, and the minister left the hospital a few days later without any further sequela.

I also want to speak to you about a blow to the sternum. This is a method that can restart the heart in the case of a cardiopulmonary arrest. This action consists in delivering a violent blow to the victim's sternum, which corresponds to a weak electric shock. That's why some people call this procedure the poor man's electric shock. In practice what happens is that in one quarter of the cases, the heart begins beating again after this blow to the chest if it is done right after the cardiac arrest. For those watching this kind of resuscitation, it is startling to see the doctor strike the patient with such force.

In beginning this chapter I spoke of certain heart illnesses such as AVNRT that can be treated using simple finger pressure on a precise point of the body. In order to understand how this type of treatment works, we need to talk about a few medical concepts. In the body there is a nerve (called the vagus nerve) that acts as a kind of brake, preventing the heart from beating too fast. By stimulating this nerve the doctor applies the brake pedal and the heart returns to its normal rhythm.

There are a number of ways of stimulating this nerve. A unilateral massage of the carotid artery for twenty seconds can only be done on young subjects whose arteries are free from atheroma. A moderate pressure on the eyeballs for thirty seconds has the same effect. It is not advisable, however, in subjects with detached retinas, glaucoma, myopia, those wearing contact lenses, or those having undergone recent eye surgery. For the record we could also mention that this is the reason that scientists have noticed a lowering of heart rate when a person rubs their eyes. There are other ways to stimulate the vagus nerve—for example by putting a finger on the uvula deep in the throat to provoke a reaction of vomiting or, less aggressively, by very quickly drinking a big glass of ice water.

In other cases a vagus nerve that is overstimulated can produce a vasovagal syncope. This illness can lead to a brief loss of consciousness caused by an insufficient amount of oxygenated blood reaching the brain. The heart rate descends too low, causing a drop in arterial pressure. The victim turns pale and passes out. A good thing to do is to raise the legs of the reclining person up at 90 degrees in order to improve irrigation of the brain while waiting for help to arrive.

Down the Wrong Way

Most often it is children or the elderly who fall victim to having something go down the wrong way. This happens during a meal when the person inadvertently swallows a foreign object such as a small bone or a fruit pit that, instead of moving down normally to the stomach, ends up blocking the air passages. When things go well the person will manage to spit out the foreign body with a strong fit of coughing. But in other cases the coughing is not enough to dislodge the intruder and the person literally suffocates. What happens is that the foreign body provokes an asphyxia by blocking the trachea.

If the person can't breathe, there is no time to lose. Help that is called at that point will likely arrive too late. The first thing to do is to place yourself beside the person, holding her upper body tilted forward and give her a series of strong slaps on the back. If that doesn't work the person will continue to suffocate. The movement of air is completely cut off, and there is no sound at all coming from the victim's mouth. She is no longer coughing at all. In this case you must change position, placing yourself behind her back, with one foot between her two feet. You need to place your fist over the pit of her stomach, under the sternum, and cover your fist with your other hand. You then make a series of very strong pulling motions, back toward yourself and up in a J-shaped movement. Someone who finds himself alone and without help can perform this procedure, called a Heimlich maneuver, in the case of asphyxia due to a foreign body. However, it cannot be done on a pregnant woman or an infant. A different procedure is required. I would add that you must never hang the person by her feet or put a finger in her mouth to provoke vomiting (because of the risk of inhaling vomit).

Stopping Bleeding or a Hemorrhage

A benign bleeding from the nose can be stopped simply by applying finger pressure. You need to begin by sitting down on a chair or on the ground. First you need to blow your nose thoroughly to dislodge possible blood clots. Then you need to bend your head forward (so the blood doesn't flow into the throat and set off vomiting). After that all you need to do is squeeze together both nostrils using your thumb and forefinger for ten minutes without stopping so clotting can take place and the bleeding can stop. Of course if only one nostril is bleeding, you only need to press closed the one side that is bleeding.

There are other cases where your fingers can save a life in stopping a hemorrhage while waiting for help to arrive. It can be a case of a limb wounded in an accident and leading to a hemorrhage that could be fatal. The action to save the person is simple. You only need to press down strongly and continuously on the wound with the fingers or the whole hand to stop the blood escaping until help can arrive. For hygienic reasons, if circumstances permit, you should place a clean cloth between your hand and the wound. Sadly it happens all too often that accident victims die surrounded by helpless bystanders. Another cause of hemorrhaging is the rupture of varicose veins in the legs. Such a break can lead to death because of the intense flow. While waiting for the emergency team to arrive, you need to get the victim to stretch out with the leg raised at a 90 degree angle to stop the hemorrhage as you press down with your hand on the spot where the blood is gushing out.

TREATING THE ENT SPECTRUM

Massaging Your Gums, the Natural Foundation of Beautiful Teeth

Healthy gums are essential to maintaining the teeth in good shape. Brushing your teeth after every meal is obvious, but daily care of the gums further improves the quality of your teeth. Grasping the gum between your thumb and index finger you can conduct a gentle and effective massage for the health of the mouth and teeth. Massage stimulates blood circulation within the gums, which is very useful especially in sensitive or painful areas. It's a simple thing to do each day that considerably reinforces the solidity of the teeth. In the summer, if you go swimming after a meal, use the sea water to conduct an aquatic massage, and you will benefit even more from the water's antiseptic effect.

Unblocking Your Nose

When your nose is blocked, your life loses some of its vitality because pleasant sensations connected to the sense of smell disappear. Air having trouble making its way through the nasal passages gives the impression that breathing is difficult, and this is interpreted as a sensation of fatigue. It can also give rise to a loss of appetite or a decrease in sexual attraction for one's spouse. The nose is also there to clean, humidify, and warm the air that is headed for the lungs.

You should know that there is a nasal cycle. On the average every three hours, one nostril partially closes, as if it is resting. Then, the other nostril partially closes, and so on, which means that you are always breathing through only one side. The length of the cycle can vary from one person to the next between one to five hours. This phenomenon corresponds to an alternating constriction and dilation in the little arteries of the nose. The blood vessels of the nasal mucous membranes receive stimuli from the sympathetic nerves that lead to a constriction of these vessels.

There is a simple thing you can do to unblock your nose. You just need to press firmly for thirty seconds with your thumb between your two eyebrows and at the same time press firmly with your tongue on the high palate. The effect is immediate and stimulates a very pleasant nasal comfort. Anatomically, this corresponds to a stimulation of specific sympathetic nerves (certain of which are situated in the sphenopalatine ganglion) that react by provoking a nasal vasoconstriction that unblocks the nose. This is like using drops to unblock your nose but without any side-effect danger, which is not always the case with some treatments.

Physiologically the nose can become blocked or unblocked spontaneously under certain circumstances. When making an effort, such as in running for example, the nose unblocks giving a sensation of well-being. Conversely, it can happen that the nose will become blocked when having sex, a phenomenon that is more developed in men who take Viagra-type medication.

The nose needs to be well humidified, and air that is too dry can sometimes lead to bleeding. Here is something pleasant you can easily try that leads to terrific nasal comfort. Before going to bed place a cotton ball dipped in water in each nostril for two minutes then take them out. This will not only bring you a very agreeable sensation of comfort, but also, according to certain specialists, this trick can reduce nighttime snoring.

Another thing—if you have water in your ears and nose after swimming, there are things you can do to drain the water away. For the nose you just need to blow your nose, and for the ears you need to bend the head forward and to the side so the water can drain away naturally.

Struggling with Dry Eyes

Almost one-third of the population suffers from dry eyes. This high level can be explained by a number of factors: urban pollution, smoking, dust, working in front of a computer screen, and age. In fact, as we age the lacrimal glands do not produce enough tears, particularly after menopause. Just having dry eyes can lead to many troublesome effects. Many people complain of sensations of having grains of sand in the eyes, a prickling or an irritation, or a particular sensitivity to cold or light. The most common symptom is that the eyes feel tired. Having tired eyes is no small thing because it can mistakenly give the impression of overall tiredness. In the evening when you're feeling worn out, one of the characteristic signs is to have a prickliness in the eyes as if they just want to close and sleep. In the middle of the day, even when someone is in good shape and wide awake, dry eyes can set off a reflex signal in the brain, as if you were already really tired.

If this is the case, it is necessary to treat dry eyes. The eyes are lubricated from the meibomian glands situated in the eyelids; these glands are designed to secrete an oily substance that protects the eye from external assault. Over time this oil becomes thicker and has trouble being exuded, which leads to the dryness.

To bring relief to your eyes, there is a simple and effective method based on two key principles: warm and massage your eyelids so that the oil, which then is more fluid, can flow. For heating I recommend using a warm, damp compress that you need to leave in place for ten minutes. Before applying to the eyes, it would be wise to test the temperature on the back of your hand. Once warmed the oil will flow out to lubricate your eyes thanks to a gentle little circular massage using your fingers. Of course you need to wash your hands before doing the eyelid massage. It is advisable to practice this little treatment once or twice a day for as long as the symptoms persist. If this is not enough, you need to consult your ophthalmologist who can prescribe various eyedrops to apply frequently during the day. I also advise that you change your pillowcases at least once a week for better hygiene, particularly of the eyelids.

I should also bring to your attention a recent Japanese study that has made clear the effect of caffeine in the production of tears. The Japanese researchers noticed that drinking four cups of coffee a day or ten cups of tea significantly reduced the frequency of having dry eyes. This observation arose from noticing that people who drank these quantities complained less of this type of pathology.

LOOKING AFTER EVERYDAY PROBLEMS

Hiccups

Hiccups often happen after a big meal or eating too fast, after laughing, coughing, or having smoked. The occasional hiccup is not serious in contrast to hiccups that keep coming back or persist and need medical attention. While there are simple little ways to stop hiccups, some people are more sensitive to one technique rather than another. That's why it's best to know about them and try them out. The simplest and best known is to drink a big glass of water. You can also try the van Wiljick maneuver, which consists of sticking out your chest as far as you can while pulling your shoulder blades toward each other and your shoulders back for ten seconds. Don't hesitate to play with the breathing rhythm by stopping the breathing briefly or engaging in very slow breathing. Ending on a funny note, I really must bring to your attention the scientific work of Dr. Odeh, who has successfully proposed a surprising treatment for curing hiccups that are resistant to various medications and the classic physical maneuvers. He stopped them with digital rectal massage. He based this on the principle that the rectum is innervated by certain nerve fibers that, when stimulated, provoke a reflex stopping of hiccups. Clearly, this very special method is suggested only for hiccups that resist all other forms of treatment.

The Side Stitch: Press Down Where It Hurts

The side stitch is a sharp pain well known to amateur athletes and sometimes even professional sports people. It is usually located under the ribs, but can also affect the collarbone, the intestines, or the stomach. It won't happen as often if you take care to begin your exercise progressively, keep well hydrated, or avoid exercising while digestion is still proceeding. Finally, there are some things you can do to get rid of the stitch when it happens. By pressing down firmly on the painful area, the release is often quick. Otherwise, you just need to bend forward while breathing out completely and the side stitch will disappear.

Knowing How to Spit

Most people often have great difficulty spitting based on cultural conditioning or embarrassment. When things are normal not spitting does not create any special problem. But when bronchial secretions are excessive, they have a tendency to give rise to a heavy, recurrent cough. Some people opt for cough syrup or antibiotics, whereas knowing when you need to spit resolves the problem easily. The technique that gives the best results is called directed expectoration. First of all you need to practice breathing in as deeply as possible. I recommend you train yourself by breathing in deeply several times in a row to increase your lung capacity. Once the air has been breathed in really fully, you need to force it out by pushing with the abdominal muscles so the air is forced out very strongly. By repeating this exercise several times, you will end up spitting and really cleaning out your lungs. I suggest that you go off by yourself so you are not embarrassed having others around. By putting this little trick into practice, you will have a terrific result: a sensation of clean lungs and a sensation of breathing fully.

Seasickness

Quite a few of us have felt that disagreeable nausea on a sea excursion, preventing us from any real enjoyment. To avoid these troubles there is a very simple exercise. Lie on your back on the floor near a wall. Place your legs vertically up against the wall for two minutes. That will quiet things down right away. And then, once you get up, keep your eyes open and stare at a point on the horizon as far away as possible without looking at the waves. Now you will enjoy the cruise.

From Aerophagia to Indigestion: The Use of Two Fingers Is All You Need

When the stomach is distended, you feel uncomfortable right away. This happens when you swallow too much air in the course of the meal. The swallowing of air is called aerophagia. We eat quickly while we talk, and all of this is washed down with carbonated beverages and without paying attention to the pressure of the air in the stomach. You are left with the sensation of a heavy meal that is going to take hours to dissipate. It's a very disagreeable sensation of discomfort and heaviness. At other times it's a question of what we simply call indigestion; the stomach doesn't manage to discharge food that has been consumed in too great a quantity. Be careful not to confuse indigestion with food poisoning, which is accompanied by diarrhea and sometimes vomiting and a fever. In the case of indigestion, it's simply a question of too much: too much food in one meal with too much grease, alcohol, side dishes, pastries, and sauces. Overwhelmed by this excess of food, the stomach is too full to empty the contents toward the intestines. All this is accompanied by a strong gastric heaviness, nausea, sometimes fatigue and headaches, feeling ill, and in all cases, a cessation of appetite.

Whether you're dealing with too much air in the stomach or indigestion, in both cases there is something simple you can do to get rid of the excess air. All you need to do is to lightly place two fingers at the bottom of the throat, which will stimulate a release of the excess air without leading to vomiting. It's an immediate release that avoids a feeling of nausea and the sensation of one's breathing feeling laden down for a whole day or night.

Chasing Cramps Away

I am only speaking here of occasional cramps in the calves that can happen sporadically and that are not serious. The cramp corresponds to a muscular contraction affecting a part of the muscle or the muscle in its entirety. Cramps happen abruptly and involuntarily. Cramps that keep coming back or cramps in other locations require medical attention. Certain factors are known to lead to cramps: dehydration, alcohol, tobacco, and cold. There are a few simple things to do to end the suffering such as simply walking, which can be enough to chase the cramp away. Another method consists of pulling back gently on the big toe while stretching the muscle. Relief is quick.

Treating Premature Ejaculation

Many men suffer from premature ejaculation. It's a disorder that spoils their lives and their partners' lives. It is defined by several criteria: a delay of less than a minute between the penetration of the penis and the ejaculation, an inability to delay the ejaculation, and the dissatisfaction of the couple. In other cases the ejaculation happens after a brief stimulation even before penetration. This disorder is very distressing to men who feel shame, anger at themselves, guilt, and loss of self-confidence.

In each case it's important to reduce the drama and start a dialogue between the partners to help resolve the issue. A premature ejaculation can happen when there is an initial sexual contact with a new partner. However, in this case, the phenomenon will disappear gradually during subsequent contacts. In other cases it's a matter of managing this disorder that leads to anxiety and frustration. Whereas sexuality is a phenomenon that generates fulfillment and relaxation, premature ejaculation, through stress and frustration, leads to a loss of all the benefits of sexuality.

There is a simple and effective method of treating premature ejaculation called the squeeze. This method was clearly defined by the American scientists Masters and Johnson, and it can help most men suffering from premature ejaculation. It is a technique of gradual reeducation conducted by the two partners. Over the course of some weeks, this technique enables the time of ejaculation to be deferred until it reaches a normal time span. At the beginning of penetration, the partner grasps the man's member at the glans with thumb on one side and the index and middle fingers on the other. The index finger needs to be placed on the head of the glans, while the middle finger is just below the head of the glans. When the man feels that he risks ejaculating, he signals to his partner who, at that moment, has to squeeze the member hard between the thumb and two fingers. This method must be conducted systematically in subsequent relations until the timing of the ejaculation satisfies the two partners. In progressively mastering ejaculation a real reeducation of male sexuality occurs. Sometimes this takes several weeks or even months. If there is no progress with this method, there are other therapeutic solutions that a doctor can prescribe.

LITERATURE

Arita, R., Y. Yanagi, N. Honda, et al. "Caffeine increases tear volume depending on polymorphisms within the adenosine A2a receptor gene and cytochrome P450 1A2." *Ophtalmology* 119(5) (2012): 972–78.

Bhavsar, A. S., S. G. Bhavsar, and S. M. Jain. "A review on recent advances in dry eye: Pathogenesis and management." *Oman Journal of Ophthalmology* 4(2) (2011): 50–56.

Blyton, F., V. Chuter, and J. Burns. "Unknotting night-time muscle cramp: A survey of patient experience, help-seeking behaviour and perceived treatment effectiveness." *Journal of Foot and Ankle Research* 5(7) (2012): doi: 10.1186/1757-1146-5-7.

Chang, F. Y., and C. L. Lu. "Hiccup: Mystery, nature and treatment." *Journal of Neurogastroenterology and Motility* 18(2) (2012): 123–30.

Iwami, T., T. Kitamura, T. Kawamura, et al. "Chest compression-only cardiopulmonary resuscitation for out-of-hospital cardiac arrest with public-access defibrillation: A nationwide cohort study." *Circulation* 126(24) (2012): 2844–51.

Krueger, W. W. "Controlling motion sickness and spatial disorientation and enhancing vestibular rehabilitation with a user-worn see-through display." *Laryngoscope* 121(suppl. 2) (2011): 17–35.

Mathers, M. J., F. Sommer, S. Degener, et al. "Premature ejaculation in urological routine practice." *Aktuelle Urologie* 44(1) (2013): 33–39; article in German.

Odeh, M., H. Bassan, and A. Oliven. "Termination of intractable hiccups with digital rectal massage." *Journal of Internal Medicine* 227(2) (1990): 145–46.

Odeh, M., and A. Oliven. "Hiccups and digital rectal massage." *Archives of Otolaryngol—Head and Neck Surgery* 119(12) (1993): 1383.

Piagkou, M., T. Demesticha, T. Troupis, et al. "The pterygopalatine ganglion and its role in various pain syndromes: From anatomy to clinical practice." *Pain Practice* 12(5) (2012): 399–412.

Smith, M. L., L. A. Beightol, J. M. Fritsch-Yelle, et al. "Valsava's maneuver revisited: A quantitative method yielding insights into human autonomic control." *American Journal of Physiology* 271(3 Pt 2) (1996): H1240–49.

Sorbara, C. "The new guidelines on cardiopulmonary resuscitation. The anesthesiologist's point of view." *Giornale Italiano di Cardiologia* 13(11) (2012): 756–53; article in Italian.

Viehweg, T. L., J. B. Roberson, and J. W. Hudson. "Epistaxis: Diagnosis and treatment." *Journal of Oral and Maxillofacial Surgery* 64(3) (2006): 511–18.

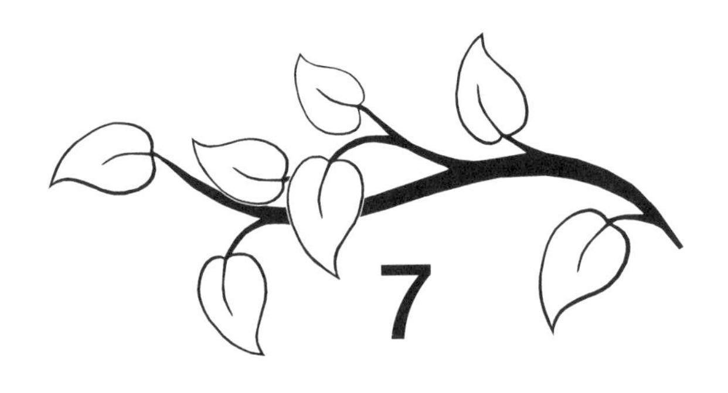

7

MOVING TOWARD SEXUAL FULFILLMENT

What is passion? It is irresistible attraction. Like that of a magnetic needle that has found its pole.

MADELEINE CHAPSAL

Judging by the surveys, subliminal advertising, and let's be honest, our daily thoughts, sexuality is at the heart of our preoccupations. And yet, it remains the source of many misunderstandings and popular beliefs, as is shown by the increasing number of consultations with sex therapists. Many of these therapists confirm that their patients often arrive completely lost in the contrast between the flood of "official" information they've been showered with and their own personal experience. In our competitive society we often mix up sexual *performance* and sexual *fulfillment*. Nevertheless, a happy sex life is the basis of good physical and mental health. It is therefore time that we set a few things straight.

TAKING BACK YOUR LIBIDO

Asking Yourself the Right Questions

The basis of sexuality rests on your libido, which we could define as energy connected to the sexual drive. For men as for women, it all begins with the first spark, the first impulse of desire attracting you to the other person. Besides the psychological factors that affect the libido, there are very real physiological and biological factors that can increase your libido or, on the contrary, decrease it. It is obvious that the libido seems stronger in a young person than in someone older, and we notice that there is a great deal of variation from one person to the next. Circumstances and the choice of partner play their role, but sometimes there are other determining factors.

A decrease in libido is a common phenomenon that can happen at any time in one's life. It makes you question your sexual desire for your partner as you attempt to understand why the attraction has diminished. Before asking metaphysical questions, you always need to investigate if your empty tank is related to a medication you are taking. In fact, a common side effect of some medications is a decrease in libido. Check it out in a standard pharmaceutical dictionary. For example, it can happen with medications that reduce cholesterol or more simply with certain contraceptive pills that lead to a decrease in desire and sexual arousal. In this case you just need to change contraceptive strategy and the libido will restart like a rocket. In short, if you are taking a treatment, even an innocuous one, read the label carefully or ask your doctor to see if your therapy is interfering with your sex life.

FOOD

Today there is a great deal of investigation into the action of certain foods on the libido. Without depending on the fairy tales and possible magic effects of such and such a food, scientifically unverified, it is especially interesting to get into new and original solutions.

Pistachios and Your Erection

Usually, when nutritional properties are discovered in a nutrient, you would need to consume astronomical quantities quite at odds with your ordinary eating habits in order to derive any benefit from it.

The example of garlic is telling: you would need to get down a whole bulb of raw garlic every day in order to derive modest benefits for your health! Even if it's a positive thing to do, someone who follows this recommendation risks being very alone because of his breath! It's not the same with pistachios: a quantity of 30 grams (1 ounce) five times a week, corresponding to 170 calories, produces results. Pistachios contain unsaturated fatty acids, fiber, and phytosterols, the cholesterol-lowering effects of which are well known. In fact, agribusiness today offers margarines and yogurts with phytosterols that support an objective lowering of cholesterol levels by 10 to 15 percent. The level of phytosterols in pistachios is 279 milligrams in 100 grams, which puts it in the top levels of foods rich in phytosterols. Pistachios are also rich in antioxidants such as anthocyanin. However, you need to know that toasting pistachios lowers their anthocyanin content (anthocyanin is a powerful antioxidant), so it is better to eat them uncooked. The other antiaging agent in pistachios is resveratrol. To round out the list of ingredients, they also contain copper, vitamin B_6, B_1, K, E, phosphorus, iron, manganese, magnesium, potassium, zinc, and selenium. It's a pity, however, that pistachios are usually salted. We consume enough salt without ingesting it pointlessly. It's best then to choose pistachios with no added ingredients.

The most surprising study on pistachios is not about the prevention of cardiovascular disease, but about sexuality. Dr. M. Aldemir in Ankara, Turkey, has demonstrated a beneficial effect on male erection, along with an improvement in blood lipid levels. He observed no side effects following this daily intake of pistachios during the three weeks that the experiment lasted.

Pomegranate, Always Pomegranate

New studies continue to uncover health benefits in pomegranates. In 2012 a study conducted in Edinburgh with sixty volunteers, both men and women, showed that drinking a daily glass of pomegranate juice produced very interesting results. The level of testosterone in the saliva rose on the average 24 percent in both men and women. As well, the study showed a slight decrease in blood pressure and an improvement in mood.

Simple Things That Work

It is clear that a sedentary lifestyle, an absence of physical exercise, tobacco, an excess of alcohol, and lack of sleep are significant factors in a marked decrease in libido in both men and women. We also need to point out that sexual prowess can be influenced negatively or positively by certain drugs and by certain foods. For example, small quantities of alcohol, like a glass of wine or champagne, diminish inhibitions thus facilitating sexual relations, while several glasses have the opposite effect, like flying your flag at half-mast. Drugs like cocaine or cannabis also lower sexual performance. Studies on rats showed that small amounts of caffeine optimize sexual relations. Here we have perhaps a new love potion so that one partner does not fall asleep too soon, forgetting the other half.

Ideally, How Long Should Sex Last? A Revolutionary Study

Sex is a powerful force, but as I said in the introduction, it is also the subject of a number of popular beliefs that can quite effectively undermine the flowering of a harmonious sexuality. How long the sexual connection should last is one of those sensitive questions that quietly troubles numerous couples. Some couples talk about it easily with each other, others say nothing, but the question is always hanging there in the background. To clear up this question, Canadian and American scientists, Doctors Corty and Guardiani, conducted a study to determine the ideal timing of a sexual connection. The time measured was from the moment of penetration into the vagina up to ejaculation. The couples afterward noted the timings and commented on the sexual enjoyment that had been felt. The results really surprised the researchers. A connection from three to seven minutes in length was determined to be just right by the couples. They also commented that a duration from seven to thirteen minutes was satisfactory. And they judged that one to two minutes was too short. The participants considered it was too long when they continued for between ten minutes and a half hour or more.

The findings in this study completely overturn the promoted stereotypes about ideal timing for sex (such as twenty minutes). So we see that longer durations did not match the pleasure criteria reported by the participants in this study—as if *too much* was fighting with *the best.* These findings are important for good sexual balance. In fact, many couples think that their performance is substandard. Such common beliefs give rise to frustration and disappointment and even lead to episodes of depression and bouts of low self-esteem. People think they're not doing very well when what they're doing is just right! Bringing the elements back to biological and physiological realities sometimes turns out to be required. Doing so helps some people stop feeling guilty and to instead enjoy the sexual connection more fully without striving for impossible performance levels. Here we have one of the keys to being happy and enjoying life.

Falling in love has now been examined in detail by scientific teams around the world. The new technology of scanners and MRI (magnetic resonance imaging) now allows us to see what is taking place in the brains of those in love. Advanced biological analyses decode the power of substances released when lovers meet or when they make love. The result is that we now know that falling in love takes only one-fifth of a second, and doing so activates at least twelve different zones inside the brain. The state of being in love leads to an immense euphoria that is comparable to the action of drugs. This natural love potion has further results as well—it is an effective antipain mechanism. Researchers at Stanford University have shown that the act of looking at your loved one reduces pain in the same way medication does but without side effects or risk of addiction.

WHEN THINGS AREN'T GOING WELL

Sexuality sometimes runs into limits and transitions from the normal to the pathological. Here are two telling examples.

Erection Problems: From Priapism to Fractured Penises

Priapism refers to a prolonged state of erection that persists more than three hours without the accompaniment of sexual stimulation. Usually, an erection is maintained by the equivalent of a hydraulic system. Blood enters through a cavernous artery that corresponds to an initial passageway. The part that can inflate and is able to provide rigidity to the erection is assured by a body of cavernous passageways. The dorsal veins of the member are there to allow the blood flow to depart—or not. These anatomical details explain why men with defective arteries have erections that are deficient in firmness and stability. When the arteries that are responsible for bringing in the blood flow needed for a good erection clog up, the diameter of the blood vessel shrinks and the blood flows less freely. The big culprits in causing the plaque that clogs up the blood flow are known: tobacco, a sedentary lifestyle, cholesterol, high blood pressure, too much sugar in the blood, and badly managed stress. It's important to realize that when a patient over forty has erection problems, his doctor needs to systematically monitor his coronary arteries to ensure that he is not at risk for a heart attack.

When a man is suffering from priapism, the doctor will look into various causes that might explain this phenomenon. For example, certain leukemias, coagulation issues, and certain medications or drugs can provoke this situation, which proves to be very painful for the victim. Each time medical teams will suggest a treatment to bring the person relief: physical exercise, having sex or repeated ejaculations, reducing the temperature of the penis, or prescription medications. In about half the cases, no cause is ever found to explain the priapism.

In recent years male sexuality has completely changed thanks to scientific progress. Even certain phenomena such as fractures of the penis are now being properly diagnosed and treated. The term *fracture* is really an overstatement since the penis does not have a central bone (except in certain mammals such as the cat). The rupture of the fibrous sheath that surrounds the body of cavernous passageways leads to violent pain. This incident occurs when the man brings too much force at the moment of penetration or in certain acrobatic positions. Treatment includes, according to the case, immobilization of the penis and sometimes even surgery followed by long periods of abstinence. Here perhaps we have an example of the old saying, "if you want to travel far, keep your vehicle in good shape."

In Good Shape till One Hundred

Progress in modern medicine ensures perfect sexuality even for elderly men. Prescriptions for testosterone creams or patches allow sexual desire to be increased in certain cases. Surgery can unblock an artery or repair a leaky vein. More and more, potent medications are being used to achieve quality erections. Treatment of premature ejaculation finally offers the possibility of resolving this inconvenient condition that certain men suffer from. Premature ejaculation is defined as a delay between penetration and ejaculation of less than one minute with no possibility of delaying the ejaculation. In spite of the efforts of both sexual partners to make the situation less dramatic, many men feel shame and feel that their virility is in question. Therapeutic progress now brings great comfort to men affected in this way.

The Female Syndrome of Continuous Genital Excitation

In women pathological excess exists as well. The syndrome of continuous genital excitation is now well known. Women who are victims of this condition present a permanent sexual excitation with the sensation of imminent orgasm. They feel a heightened sensitivity in the areas of the clitoris, vagina, labia majora, and sometimes the perineum. This syndrome manifests in episodes that can last from several hours to several days, and orgasms do not relieve someone suffering from this condition. Research has attempted to explain the condition. A Dutch team has just discovered a link to "restless leg syndrome" that opens a pathway for the analysis of this disorder. Other scientists are investigating origins that could be linked to hormonal disturbances.

THE SECRETS OF THE FRENCH KISS

The French are known throughout the whole world for the famous French kiss—a long, deep, and loving kiss, mouth to mouth and using the tongue. This kiss is a subtle message for transmitting feelings that are hard to express in words. It's an exchange that activates various senses such as taste, smell, and touch. This practice, which astonishes a lot of Anglo-Saxons, is a real gem of French cultural heritage.

The Biochemistry of the Kiss: An Alchemy of Well-Being

Scientific research now allows us to understand exactly what mechanisms take place in a kiss. Studies were done on heterosexual student couples who were asked to kiss for fifteen minutes. Analyses of saliva and blood were conducted to investigate hormonal substances secreted during the experiment. The research identified three stages:

- Saliva participates in the increase of sexual desire since it contains testosterone. Testosterone, as much in men as in women, sets in motion a stronger sexual drive. This is the sexual dimension of the kiss.
- As a second stage you have the secretion of dopamine, which could be termed the pleasure hormone. This is the romantic dimension of the kiss.

- Finally, as a third stage, the secretion of oxytocin, the bonding and well-being hormone, provides the dimension of the participants becoming *a couple* after the first kiss.

The results underscored that the kiss played a role as an unconscious means of evaluating the partner. In practice about 60 percent of men and women state that, after the first kiss, they stopped pursuing a relationship with that partner.

A kiss acts like a trigger that liberates hormone flow, the effects of which are excellent for health. Among these are the release of small quantities of endorphins. These molecules, which are close to the composition of morphine, when released in small quantities and without danger to your health, produce a sensation of gentle euphoria and relaxation. To round out this hormonal fireworks display, we need to mention dopamine. Dopamine is a neurotransmitter of pleasure and reward that the brain releases during an experience that it determines is beneficial. It is also interesting to note that dopamine is a component in various processes of addiction such as with drugs. I far prefer being addicted to kissing, which is natural. You only need one passionate kiss that lasts at least twenty seconds to release this hormonal cataclysm. Certain scientists, such as evolutionary psychologist Gordon Gallup of the University of Albany and Rutgers University anthropologist Helen Fisher, have suggested that male saliva contains tiny quantities of testosterone that, when transmitted to a woman, boost her libido.

Kissing and Massage: Effective Anti-Stress Agents

By providing this cocktail of hormones, the kiss acts as a powerful and natural anti-stress agent. It is important to note that saliva also contains pheromones, especially in men. Scientific studies have shown that pheromones modify the emotional state of the female partner when she receives saliva from a man. In studying the hormonal changes in men and women following a prolonged kiss, a lowering of the cortisol level was observed; cortisol could be called a biological stress marker. In practice then, the kiss is a powerful anti-stress agent and presents no danger, unlike some medications. The pleasure that is generated can be habit forming, but there are no contraindications and no side effects. This would lead one to assume that the French, who are the highest consumers in the world of anxiolytics (anti-stress agents) don't kiss enough!

Massage is also a powerful anti-stress agent. We need to highlight the work of Dr. Beate Ditzen in Zurich. She tested two different methods of psychological support. To do this she brought together couples where the wife had to speak publically, which is a stressor. In the first group the husband reassured her with gentle and reassuring words, and in the second group the husband practiced a ten-minute massage on her neck and shoulders. The results showed that only the group who had been massaged benefited from the anti-stress effect with a lowering of cortisol level in the saliva and a slower heart rate.

Being Apart for a Week Is Not Good for Your Health

The work of a team at the University of Utah investigated the impact that a separation of four to seven days had on couples. They observed that a significant number of couples showed signs of stress—among the factors was a poor quality of sleep, which showed up biologically as an increase in cortisol. Heart rates also increased. It was found that if one partner had numerous external professional or social contacts, the stress was lessened. In contrast, the presence of children in the home was not a determining factor in stress reduction.

INCREASING YOUR POWERS OF SEDUCTION

The Power of a Look: Four Fateful Minutes

Oscar Wilde was quite right in claiming that beauty is in the eye of the beholder. A scientific study conducted in the United States has recently shown the incredible power that can be set in motion by the intensity of a simple look. Dr. Arthur Aron found that looking intently at a partner made a decisive impact on the activation of feeling in that partner. In conducting these scientific studies, he brought together men and women who were not acquainted with each other beforehand. He then arranged them in couples by randomly choosing partners for each one of them. For the first half hour, he asked each person in the just-formed couples to speak about his or her day-to-day life including all sorts of detail, even intimate things. At the end of thirty minutes, he required that the couples not say a word and that they look into each other's eyes in complete silence for exactly four minutes. The majority of participants experienced, following this lengthy look into each other's eyes, a deep attraction to the partner who had been a stranger to them a half an hour before. In fact, six months later, two of the couples in this study got married.

I must say that the four minutes intrigued me. Especially when I discovered that trained hypnotists can put subjects into a state of sleep in only five seconds. I looked for explanations among practitioners who use hypnosis in their practice. Hypnosis is a technique that has been in use for a long time. Early on, in 1878, at the Salpêtrière Hospital in Paris, Dr. Charcot used it to treat patients who showed manifestations of hysteria. Hypnotists consider that there is an unknown power in the look that allows them to plunge the subject into a state between wakefulness and sleep. By the way, this state is characterized by specific wavelengths clearly visible on an electroencephalogram reading. This borderline state between wakefulness and sleep is a moment of vulnerability during which defense mechanisms are lowered. Thus, like a stroke of lightning, it opens a passageway into the unconscious.

From a technical point of view, hypnotists consider that anyone can learn to use the hypnotic power of a fixed look. You just need to practice. They particularly stress the ability to stare fixedly, the capacity to not blink the eyelids, and the importance of the diameter of the pupils. With the pupils there are two situations. Having dilated pupils is called mydriasis (the opposite, when pupils contract is called myosis). Pupil dilation can be related to a particular physiological state, to the taking of certain medications, or to illness. In practice, consuming alcohol or drugs can provoke this dilation, but so can the natural adaptation of the eyes when moving from light into darkness. An intense emotion such as exchanging a kiss can also provoke mydriasis. Coming back to everyday life, don't hesitate to bring your look into play; its power is much greater than your words. Looking fixedly into your partner's eyes, with your eyes wide open and not looking elsewhere, will bring you surprising results.

Daring to Discover Your True Sexual Orientation

Following the example of Hippocrates who wisely said, "As with the eyes, so with the body," a distinguished team of scientists at Cornell University subjected 325 volunteers, men and women, to the viewing of very erotic videos. Using infrared lenses they measured the pupil dilation in real time as a function of the various scenes in the films. They determined that heterosexual men's pupils dilated upon seeing women; homosexual men's pupils dilated upon seeing men. Conversely, women's pupils dilated as much for scenes that involved men as for scenes that involved women. Lesbian women showed responses similar to heterosexual men.

The interesting feature of this study is that it showed the real desire that a man or a woman experienced as separate from social conventions, taboos, or forbidden activities. Men or women can have strong attractions toward the same sex without ever daring to express them, based on their education or their circumstances. Not feeling right in themselves, they risk developing states of depression or modes of compensation such as overuse of tobacco, alcohol, or food. The principle of *know thyself* is the foundation of a life that expands into feeling good at every moment. When people build a life that contradicts their own deep nature, they will do nothing but lie to themselves and to those around them. Living "as if" casts a gray shadow on life and leads to immense, unexplained fatigue. We need, therefore, to pay homage to the volunteers in this scientific study, which was conducted with great care, for the courage it must have taken for the participants to discover and reveal their own deep tendencies.

The True Power of Tears

Female tears send specific signals to men. In order to investigate these signals, researchers at the Weizman Institute of Science in Israel studied the effect of women's tears on men. They noted that the tears brought on a lowering of sexual excitement and desire in the men. In conducting this study the Israeli researchers made the women cry by showing them sad films. The scientists collected the tears, then had the men sniff them. The men didn't know what they were smelling. The experiment showed that following contact with the scent of tears, the men had a lowering of testosterone and of sexual desire. An MRI exam confirmed the data by showing a distinct lessening of activity in the affected cerebral zones. A woman crying releases the emission of chemical signals that provoke a drop in testosterone in men. Testosterone is a hormone that increases men's desire for women. British researchers, by the way, have shown that men's attraction for female faces is directly linked to their level of testosterone. The higher the level of this hormone, the stronger the desire. Female tears act like an extinguisher of male desire through the release of olfactory signals. For the moment the chemical analysis of the components has not been determined, and studies have not yet been conducted on the signals in male tears. Some women should perhaps think twice before crying in order to be seductive, because the effect risks being the opposite of what they intend.

The Art of Persuasion

Some hypnotists work with techniques of persuasion by triggering very specific mechanisms. They restrain themselves by speaking as little as possible and by sustaining a distant and mysterious attitude. While maintaining an attitude of deep calm, they appear completely disinterested, waiting a few interminable seconds before clasping an outstretched hand. The hypnotist remains as much as possible in the background, immobile, while at the same time encouraging the subject to let go as much as possible. Saying nothing, or very little, puts the critical mind to sleep and unconsciously pushes subjects to engage as much as possible in making themselves liked by the one holding the power, who never gets to the point of seduction.

Being more seductive in order to overcome what seems impossible means beginning to submit to the power of the person who refuses to smile or who acts as though you don't matter to them. It's the opposite of seduction that attracts the other person. This is typically the case in certain young women who are not attracted in the least by men who flatter them too much; instead they prefer to dream of one day becoming the girlfriend of some rustic and unsophisticated country boy. Seduction in this case is based on emphasizing what he lacks or on highlighting what he doesn't have in order to attract more. What's missing then shakes the subject's foundations by highlighting her own limitations, and that immediately brings to the surface all the conscious and unconscious complexes that might explain to the subject why the hypnotist is not being seductive toward her: feeling too short or too tall, too fat or too thin, too distant or daddy's darling, too old or too young.

Hundreds of variations exist and constitute the triggers of individual neuroses. Once activated these mechanisms provide all the means required for seduction. The individual who knows these techniques, techniques I would call anti-seduction, becomes a masterful seducer. However, this requires great self-mastery and a talent for observation that has been honed and sharpened. This behavior goes against a person's natural reflexes, which consist of seducing in an automatic way using smiles and compliments. Acting as an anti-seducer requires one to hold back in order to feel out a situation and, above all, to concentrate on listening to the other person. Listening is an essential element. Concentrating on what is said to you without thinking of what you might reply requires a high degree of concentration. Very few people really know how to listen; most people talk to hear themselves talk and no one really listens to what the other person is saying. The individual who discovers active listening to others gains true power over them, like the psychoanalyst with her patient or the priest with his faithful parishioner.

LITERATURE

Aldemir, M., E. Okulu, S. Neşelioğlu, et al. "Pistachio diet improves erectile function parameters and serum lipid profiles in patients with erectile dysfunction." *International Journal of Impotence Research* 23(1) (2011): 32–38.

Aron, A., H. Fisher, D. J. Mashek, et al. "Reward, motivation, and emotion systems associated with early-stage intense romantic love." *Journal of Neurophysiology* 94(1) (2005): 327–37.

Aron, E. N., A. Aron, and J. Jagiellowicz. "Sensory processing sensitivity: A review in the light of the evolution of biological responsivity." *Personality and Social Psychology Review* 16(3) (2012): 262–82.

Bartels, A., and S. Zeki. "The neural basis of romantic love." *Neuroreport* 11(17) (2000): 3829–34.

Bartels, A., and S. Zeki. "The neural correlates of maternal and romantic love." *NeuroImage* 21 (2004): 1155–66.

Basler, A. J. "Pilot study investigating the effects of Ayurvedic Abhyanga massage on subjective stress experience." *Journal of Alternative and Complementary Medicine* 17(5) (2011): 435–40.

Bianchi-Demicheli, F., S. T. Grafton, and S. Ortigue. "The power of love on the human brain." *Social Neuroscience* 1(2) (2006): 90–103.

Cambron, J. A., J. Dexheimer, and P. Coe. "Changes in blood pressure after various forms of therapeutic massage: A preliminary study." *Journal of Alternative and Complementary Medicine* 12(1) (2006): 65–70.

Campo, J., M. A. Perea, J. del Romero, et al. "Oral transmission of HIV, reality or fiction? An update." *Oral Diseases* 12(3) (2006): 219–28.

Cohen, M. S., D. C. Shugars, and S. A. Fiscus. "Limits on oral transmission of HIV-1." *Lancet* 356(9226) (2000): 272.

Corty, E. W. "Perceived ejaculatory latency and pleasure in different outlets." *Journal of Sexual Medicine* 5(11) (2008): 2694–2702.

Corty, E. W., and J. M. Guardiani. "Canadian and American sex therapist's perceptions of normal and abnormal ejaculatory latencies: How long should intercourse last?" *Journal of Sexual Medicine* 5(5) (2008): 1251–56.

Cox, S. W., E. M. Rodriguez-Gonzalez, V. Booth, and B. M. Eley. "Secretory leukocyte protease inhibitor and its potential interactions with elastase and cathepsin B in gingival crevicular fluid and saliva from patients with chronic periodontitis." *Journal of Periodontal Research* 41(5) (2006): 477–85.

Crane, J. D., D. I. Ogborn, C. Cupido., et al. "Massage therapy attenuates inflammatory signaling after exercise-induced muscle damage." *Science Translational Medicine* 4(119) (2012): doi: 10.1126/scitranslmed.3002882.

De Boer, A., E. M. van Buel, and G. J. Ter Horst. "Love is more than just a kiss: A neurobiological perspective on love and affection." *Neuroscience* 201 (2012): 114–124.

Denison, F. C., V. E. Grant, A. A. Calder, and R. W. Kelly. "Seminal plasma components stimulate interleukin-8 and interleukin-10 release." *Molecular Human Reproduction* 5(3) (1999): 220–26.

Diamond, L. M., A. M. Hicks, and K. D. Otter-Henderson. "Every time you go away: Changes in affect, behavior, and physiology associated with travel-related separations from romantic partners." *Journal of Personality and Social Psychology* 95(2) (2008): 385–403.

Diamond, L. M., and K. Wallen. "Sexual minority women's sexual motivation around the time of ovulation." *Archives of Sexual Behavior* 40(2) (2011): 237–46.

Ditzen, B., I. D. Neumann, G. Bodenmann, et al. "Effects of different kinds of couple interaction on cortisol and heart rate responses to stress in women." *Psychoneuroendocrinology* 32(5) (2007): 565–74.

Doumas, S., A. Kolokotronis, and P. Stefanopoulos. "Anti-inflammatory and antimicrobial roles of secretory leukocyte protease inhibitor." *Infection and Immunity* 73(3) (2005): 1271–74.

Emanuele, E., P. Politi, M. Bianchi, et al. "Raised plasma nerve growth factor levels associated with early-stage romantic love." *Psychoneuroendocrinology* 31(3) (2006): 288–94.

Forest, C. P., H. Padma-Nathan, and H. R. Liker. "Efficacy and safety of pomegranate juice on improvement of erectile dysfunction in male patients with mild to moderate erectile dysfunction: A randomized placebo-controlled, double-blind, crossover study." *International Journal of Impotence Research* 19(6) (2007): 564–67.

Garcia, F. D., and F. Thibaut. "Sexual addictions." *American Journal of Drug and Alcohol Abuse* 36(5) (2010): 254–60.

Gelstein, S., Y. Yeshurun, L. Rozenkrantz, et al. "Human tears contain a chemosignal." *Science* 331(6014) (2011): 226–30.

Goertz, C. H., R. H. Grimm, K. Svendsen, and G. Grandits. "Treatment of Hypertension with Alternative Therapies (THAT) Study: A randomized clinical trial." *Journal of Hypertension* 20(10) (2002): 2063–68.

Grewen, K. M., B. J. Anderson, S. S. Girdler, and K. C. Light. "Warm partner contact is related to lower cardiovascular reactivity." *Behavioral Medicine* 29(3) (2003): 123–30.

Grewen, K. M., S. S. Girdler, and K. C. Light. "Relationship quality: Effects on ambulatory blood pressure and negative affect in a biracial sample of men and women." *Blood Pressure Monitoring* 10(3) (2005): 117–24.

Hardestam, J., L. Petterson, C. Ahlm, et al. "Antiviral effect of human saliva against hantavirus." *Journal of Medical Virology* 80(12) (2008): 2122–26.

Hendrie, C. A., and G. Brewer. "Kissing as an evolutionary adaptation to protect against human cytomegalovirus-like teratogenesis." *Medical Hypotheses* 74(2) (2010): 222–24.

Jefferson, L. L. "Exploring effects of therapeutic massage and patient teaching in the practice of diaphragmatic breathing on blood pressure, stress, and anxiety in hypertensive African-American women: An intervention study." *Journal of National Black Nurses Association* 21(1) (2010): 17–24.

Kimata, H. "Kissing selectively decreases allergen-specific IgE production in atopic patients." *Journal of Psychosomatic Research* 60(5) (2006): 545–47.

Kort, H. I., J. B. Massey, C. W. Elsner, et al. "Impact of body mass index values on sperm quantity and quality." *Journal of Andrology* 27(3) (2006): 450–52.

Maloney, J. M., M. D. Chapman, and S. H. Sicherer. "Peanut allergen exposure through saliva: Assessment and interventions to reduce exposure." *Journal of Allergy and Clinical Immunology* 118(3) (2006): 719–24.

Moeini, M., M. Givi, Z. Ghasempour, and M. Sadeghi. "The effect of massage therapy on blood pressure of women with pre-hypertension." *Iranian Journal of Nursing and Midwifery Research* 16(1) (2011): 61–70.

Olney, C. M. "The effect of therapeutic back massage in hypertensive persons: A preliminary study." *Biological Research for Nursing* 7(2) (2005): 98–105.

Ortigue, S., F. Bianchi-Demicheli, N. Patel, et al. "Neuroimaging of love: fMRI meta-analysis evidence toward new perspectives in sexual medicine." *Journal of Sexual Medicine* 7(11) (2010): 3541–52.

Pfaffe, T., J. Cooper-White, P. Beyerlein, et al. "Diagnostic potential of saliva:

Current state and future applications." *Clinical Chemistry* 57(5) (2011): 675–87.

Rieger, G., and R. C. Savin-Williams. "The eyes have it: Sex and sexual orientation differences in pupil dilation patterns." *PloS One* 7(8) (2012): doi: 10.1371/journal.pone.0040256.

Sharkey, D. J., K. P. Tremellen, M. J. Jasper, et al. "Seminal fluid induces leukocyte recruitment and cytokine and chemokine mRNA expression in the human cervix after coitus." *Journal of Immunology* 188(5) (2012): 2445–54.

Shugars, D. C., S. P. Sweet, D. Malamud, et al. "Saliva and inhibition of HIV-1 infection: Molecular mechanisms." *Oral Diseases* 8(suppl. 2) (2002): 169–75.

Smith, M., N. Geffen, T. Alasbali, et al. "Digital ocular massage for hypertensive phase after Ahmed valve surgery." *Journal of Glaucoma* 19(1) (2010): 11–14.

Waldinger, M. D., and D. H. Schweitzer. "Persistent genital arousal disorder in 18 Dutch women: Part. II. A syndrome clustered with restless legs and overactive bladder." *Journal of Sexual Medicine* 6(2) (2009): 482–97.

———. "Retarded ejaculation in men: An overview of psychological and neurobiological insights." *World Journal of Urology* 23(2) (2005): 76–81.

Waldinger, M. D., A. P. van Gils, H. P. Ottervanger, et al. "Persistent genital arousal disorder in 18 Dutch women: Part I. MRI, EEG, and transvaginal ultrasonography investigations." *Journal of Sexual Medicine* 6(2) (2009) 474–81.

Welling, L. L., B. C. Jones, L. M. DeBruine, et al. "Men report stronger attraction to femininity in women's faces when their testosterone levels are high." *Hormones and Behavior* 54(5) (2008): 703–8.

Werner, C., T. Fürster, T. Widmann, et al. "Physical exercise prevents cellular senescence in circulating leukocytes and in the vessel wall." *Circulation* 120(24) (2009): 2438–47.

Wiesner, J., and A. Vilcinskas. "Antimicrobial peptides: The ancient arm of the human immune system." *Virulence* 1(5) (2010): 440–64.

Younger, J., A. Aron, S. Parke, et al. "Viewing pictures of romantic partner reduces experimental pain: Involvement of neural reward systems." *PLoS One* 5(10) (2010): e13309.

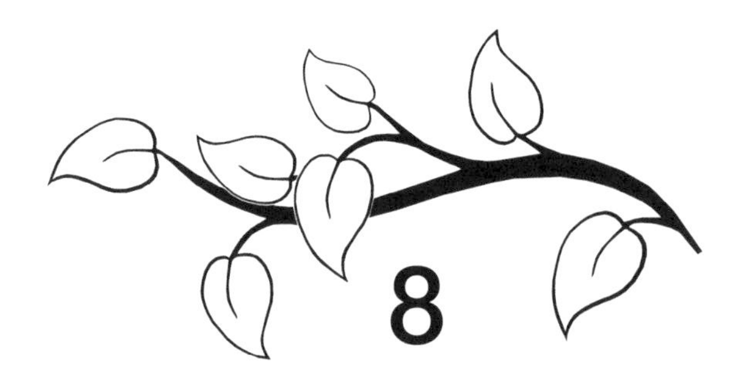

8

ELIMINATING STRESS AND DEPRESSION

Start by changing yourself if you want to change the life around you.

GANDHI

It's no secret that the French are great lovers of anxiolytics and antidepressants. According to the French Health Products Safety Agency, France is the second greatest consumer of anxiolytics in Europe and at least one French person in five takes them.* These pharmaceuticals, mass produced in the 1960s, have certainly allowed many patients to be healed and have finally meant that these very real pathologies are now taken seriously—such as chronic stress or depression. But every coin has two sides. Putting yourself in a chemical straightjacket can be harmful in the long run because these medications come with numerous undesirable side effects: addiction, memory loss, reduced libido, inability to confront the events of life. Here, too, there are simple and natural preventive means for keeping your mental processes in shape, such as the practice of happiness (yes, happiness can be learned!) and meditation.

*Source: Afssaps (Agence Française de Sécurité Sanitaire des Produits de Santé [French Health Products Safety Agency]), 2012.

BRINGING STRESS TO A HALT

Setting Something Straight

Here are phrases you hear again and again: "I'm stressed," "My job is stressing me out," "My kids are stressful!" In short, stress comes in all flavors. Numerous books and articles have been devoted to this disease of the century, and I'm not going to repeat here what you've doubtless read a ton of times. I simply want to remind you of a few points that you need to keep in mind before getting into natural healing techniques.

Burnout or the Outer Limits of Stress

When your body is subjected to repeated, uncontrolled stress, it becomes exhausted and no longer knows how to react. This is the final stage of stress, and it can be disastrous for your health. There is a great deal of talk these days about burnout or the syndrome of professional exhaustion—this is a typical case of prolonged stress occasioned by professional activities. The stressing agents can belong to different orders of stress: negative environmental factors, pressure from top management, unattainable goals, incompatibility with one's private life, excessive travel time, or overcommitment to the job.

At first the body reacts as if it can manage the stress. It's hard, but you think you can manage and you don't pay too much attention. In the following phase it's like a car motor that has run out of gas, but you keep trying to move on by making huge efforts. And then one day—complete breakdown; you're no longer able to get out of bed to go to work and suffering is at such a level that you just stop working. Then there is guilt, plummeting self-worth, and even depression. As you can see stress needs to be taken very seriously and dealt with wisely to avoid such dead ends.

Stress is a normal reaction of the organism that allows it to respond to agreeable or disagreeable stimulation from the outside. Under the effect of stress, your body produces adrenaline to push you to act, as well as various hormones (endorphins, cortisol) to allow you to meet these situations and make decisions. So if you never underwent any stress, you would be like some kind of reptile! Unfortunately, when we are overstimulated (too much activity, increased competition), overchallenged (things going wrong, frustration, pressures at work), or just tired, the body no longer has a chance to relax between two phases of stress. It stops managing exterior stimuli and starts eating away at itself with a procession of unpleasant manifestations: anxiety, psychosomatic illnesses, feeling out of sorts, psychological disturbances, insomnia, irritability, and nutritional disturbances. Here is where you need to take action—before it's too late.

Without having recourse to medication or magic potions, there are totally free and extremely simple means of reducing your stress. One thing is certain: it is impossible to eliminate stress from our lives; we have to learn to live with it.

PHYSICAL MEANS

Touch

Americans often hug each other as a form of greeting when they meet as couples or friends. The hug is a sort of affectionate hello that consists of taking the other person in your arms with a light squeeze. It produces a physical intimacy as the arms wrap around the neck or rest affectionately on the back of your partner. Based on the circumstances it can be an expression of friendship, love, or at least companionship and familiarity. It's a romantic form of exchange in the modern world, a vector of emotion, happiness, and human warmth—a strong signal of welcoming and opening.

In India a woman by the name of Amma has conferred this hug to more than thirty million individuals. This woman, whom many consider to be an incarnation of divinity, is known for using this hug to bestow numerous benefits upon the person who receives it. In those moments she transmits *darshan*—a powerful spiritual energy. I observed a ceremony where Amma practiced this greeting with hundreds of the faithful, and I, too, had the privilege of being taken in her arms. It is a unique experience that is charged with emotion. You have the impression of immense positive energy surrounding you, protecting you, and calming you. It amounts to a kind of flashback in order to return to one's foundations, to what is essential, to once again find one's own authentic path. It was at that precise moment that I understood what I had seen on the faces of the faithful after this contact—a prodigious feeling of calm and serenity.

A team of researchers in the psychiatry department at the University of North Carolina has decoded for the first time the benefits of a hug. To do that they conducted several studies, which all came to the same conclusions. In this investigation they assembled fifty-nine women ranging in age from twenty to forty-nine who had been with the same partner for six months whether they were married or not. They then compared one group who never received a hug to a group who received repeated hugs from their partners. In doing this they discovered that the hugs increased the secretion of oxytocin—the hormone that could be called the coupling and well-being hormone. This secretion generated a reduced heart rate, lower blood pressure, and a reduction in stress.

Massage

In the context of close contact, massage is often cited as a source of well-being. It contributes to serenity and relaxation by creating a calming world. It reduces stress while at the same time promoting a better connection to the body and to the mind. Going for a massage is strong indication that you've decided to look after yourself. Until 2012 there was a lack of serious studies that objectively demonstrated the effect of massage on health. The work of Dr. Mark Tarnopolsky of McMaster University in Ontario, Canada, has recently shown the anti-inflammatory effects of massage, accompanied by elements of regeneration and recuperation at a muscular level. Dr. Tarnopolsky's team worked with a group of sports enthusiasts who, after significant workouts, were treated to a long massage on just one of their legs. The researchers then took small muscle samples before and after the workout on the massaged and nonmassaged legs. The results were astonishing. The analyses uncovered a marked anti-inflammatory effect in the massaged legs as if an anti-inflammatory medication had been locally injected. They also demonstrated an increase in the number of mitochondria in the cells, indicating that the efficiency of the muscles had improved. Mitochondria contribute to the production of cellular energy. The researchers even managed to understand the biological mechanism underlying these beneficial effects. In fact, when the masseur's hand exerts pressure on the skin, this action provokes a series of biological reactions. Receptors located on the cellular surfaces initiate messages that activate molecules called kinases that, in turn, activate specific genes that are known to intervene in the struggle against inflammation.

The team of Daniel Fletcher, professor of bioengineering at Berkeley and faculty scientist at the Berkeley Lab, has performed an unusual experiment. They subjected cancerous cells of a breast tumor to a pressure of 0.05 bar (equivalent to the pressure felt under 50 centimeters, or 20 inches, of water) for a period of thirty minutes. Contrary to all expectations one-third of the cancerous cells ceased proliferating and returned to a normal form that they retained after the pressure was removed. They began communicating with each other normally. This opens an unexpected avenue of research related to the placing of manual pressure on the human body.

The Protection of a Smile

Even if you force yourself to smile, you will be helping yourself. This is the result of recent research done by psychologists Tara Kraft and Sarah Pressman at the University of Kansas. The study was done with 169 volunteers who were subjected to stressful situations. In the group that was forced to smile by holding chopsticks in their mouths in a prescribed manner, the doctors noticed that those volunteers were distinctly less sensitive to stress. This observation was based on a reduction in the heart rate provoked by the smiles that were repeated during stress. Stress is very harmful to your health. It underlies numerous pathologies such as cardiac disease.

However, as we have said, it is impossible to live in an environment without stress, and it would even be dangerous to do so because the organism needs a minimum of daily stress to marshal its defenses. We have permanent access to the strength needed to combat stressful situations. A forced smile immediately lowers the stress level, which is good for our cells. If the stress is coming from the person facing you, repeatedly adopt a forced smile. You will relax, and conversely, you will observe an increase in stress in the person you are speaking with. Test it out. If you smile spontaneously and naturally, that works just as well but it's not as easy to control.

Don't hesitate to smile as often as you can. Smiles generate positive waves around you and create an impression of success, making you more attractive. You will look more rested and younger. Moreover, the good mood that the smiles generate is contagious. Try thinking of something sad or negative, and smile at the same time. Then you will understand the power the smile has to protect you.

LEARN TO LIBERATE YOURSELF MENTALLY

Silencing Our Mental Policeman

In May 1968 you could see the saying, "The cop is inside you" written everywhere on the walls of Paris. It is still true today, but more insidiously. The overly authoritarian policeman, parent, or professor are easy-to-spot targets that then can be fought, ignored, or left behind. However, when the inner enemy looks like an ally, a friend, or the image of what one should be to belong to a group, the struggle is not so simple and stands in the way of life by blocking possibilities. Many people have an immense potential stored within themselves that they are never going to use—childhood dreams, not the least shred of which ever penetrate into their adult lives. It's all those things that distance us from who we really are, from our center of gravity, or quite simply from happiness. Early on in life messages get transmitted in this direction with more or less intensity. With childhood encouragement to "eat up to make Mommy happy" and "finish your plate" how many people, now adult, finish their plates even though the food was not good at all and they're no longer hungry?

Learn to Say No!

Here's a sketch of a few little suggestions for learning how to liberate yourself:

- Decline an invitation if you're feeling too tired.
- Don't wear the jacket that everyone says you look great in if you're not comfortable wearing it.
- At night when you're dead tired and someone offers you a last drink, go home.
- When the telephone rings and it's not a good moment, don't pick up. If it's urgent you will always find out about it.
- Don't accept that promotion if you feel, deep down, that you are not capable or that it doesn't suit you.

Subconsciously, they have the impression that they will be less loved if they don't conform to the rules. Learning to not finish your plate by listening to what you're really feeling is the first step toward happiness. It is very difficult to free oneself from the subconscious inner look of the kind person, but it's the price of freedom. In other cases certain people begin to drink, to smoke, or take drugs in order to belong to a group that provides them with an identity. But as they do they are gradually destroying themselves and shortening their lives. This issue can also involve the choice of spouse by selecting someone who corresponds to what is good for one's parents, friends, or worse—images of stars in a television series. This is how it starts and how it leads to ruined lives, unhappy children, and a never-ending sensation of things going badly. The choice of a profession can work in the same way: you choose a profession based on your social group and not on your own deep aspirations.

Facing Reality to Break Your Chains

To be happy you have to know how to break visible and invisible chains so that your life corresponds to the person living it. It's a difficult road and sometimes requires help because we don't always see what is restricting us in spite of ourselves. In difficult cases psychoanalysis can allow us to free ourselves and find out who we really are. I regret that in France psychoanalysis is still taboo. For many people seeing a psychoanalyst means you think you're crazy. This is a big mistake since the technique of psychoanalysis brings to light blocking mechanisms that have been there since childhood, acting like brakes that interfere with the motor of life. It often requires help to find them, and it is difficult to dislodge them by oneself—a little like a surgeon who might try to operate on himself all alone.

Defenses

Psychological defenses make things particularly difficult. In order to imagine what defenses are like, think of a very painful, sore spot on your arm. If someone tries to touch it, even very lightly, you will push them away—forcefully and reflexively. When you find yourself again faced with the same situation, you will be on your guard and you will react even more quickly and strongly. Psychoanalysts know perfectly well about these defense mechanisms. That is why they approach sensitive points prudently as if they were defusing a bomb, and thus, the analysis can sometimes last several years. A thousand precautions are taken to arrive at the goal. This also explains why we often violently push away those close to us who tell us the truth. They may be right, but without knowing it they are pushing on a defense mechanism that neutralizes their efforts. Someone who is impartial and is outside the affective context will be able to make more progress. You can understand why the college of physicians recommends that doctors not treat their own family, that a surgeon not operate on a family member, and that a psychoanalyst not engage in therapy with close family. Defusing a defense mechanism is long and difficult work, but it is worth the effort; it can restore freedom to those who have lost it.

Transference

Transference is another difficulty that sometimes happens during psychoanalysis. Here I am speaking of the arising of feeling between the analyst and patient. For example, the psychoanalyst may, at a given moment, represent the father or the mother. This affective transference will make progress difficult and tends to bring into play the mechanism whereby the patient tries to convince the other person, the psychoanalyst, of something. Trying to convince in this way means trying to appear to be what, in reality, you are not. Wanting to show what you think is the best side of yourself is not at all the same as showing yourself as you are. It amounts to building roads to nowhere in order to confuse the other person and then convince her. You then risk doing all you can to live up to the image that you have created in your effort to convince the other person. This amounts to locking yourself up in a prison, repeating the same scenario as if from a stage play, and abolishing what one really is. It's a loss of authenticity.

To free yourself you absolutely must not fall into any mechanism of trying to convince someone of something; on the contrary, you must dare to appear as you are. This is certainly a risk in psychoanalysis: by revealing individuals to themselves as they really are, they become strangers to their own life. The danger of a break, be it affective, social, or professional, is great when people decide to cut the invisible ties that are blocking them. Delicate choices for sure, but this is also the price of freedom and happiness.

AVOIDING FEELING DOWN

As with stress *feeling down* is part of our daily vocabulary, and we have all experienced it at certain times in our lives. Feeling down is characterized by emotional and physical fatigue, brooding, and having a tendency to see the glass as half empty. You have less get up and go, things hold little or no interest for you, and any activity seems difficult. Feeling down can happen at difficult moments in life, or even just when everything seems dull and ordinary. You might think—wrongly—that you are depressed just because you are not happy all the time and the days and weeks are full of changing moods. Feeling down is different from depression, which is characterized by the same symptoms but more serious ones (everything slows down and the person has no interest in anything) and it lasts continuously for more than two weeks. Clearly you need to consult a doctor if you or someone close to you is in this state. Feeling down on the other hand does not last and can be addressed using natural techniques.

Cultivating Happiness

All recent research indicates that happiness is a guarantee of longevity with good health. Happy people have longer telomeres. Telomeres are little end pieces of our chromosomes that gradually shorten as we age. The more the telomeres shorten, the greater the incidence of diseases such as cancer, Alzheimer's, or cardiovascular disease. It turns out that people of the same age who have longer telomeres are people who are happier. It's simply a question of knowing how to be happy; many books are published on this topic, offering you a thousand and one reasons for seeing life positively. For now happiness is not taught in schools, which is a pity. However, there is one exception: An American university has offered courses in happiness, and it is not just any university because we're talking about Harvard, a most prestigious one. This course fills the classroom to capacity. When you take into account that the cost of college courses is far from negligible, you realize the enormous interest the students must have for this new discipline.

Yes, happiness can be learned, and getting to happiness is not necessarily obvious. It depends more on a state of mind and on a particular outlook on life than on material circumstances. Certain people are happy with three times nothing, and others, wielding immense fortunes and living in loving and stable families, find themselves in a state of chronic depression. Some people seem to enjoy a mysterious alchemy that gives them immense strength and well-being. External events do not overtake them, and they have an impressive power available to them: the ability to be happy in most of life's circumstances. However, in order to access this state that completely changes what life deals out to you, you need to keep to a certain path. I will provide you with a few tools here that I hope will contribute to helping you find your way to lasting happiness.

Unstable Equilibriums

Think of men and women who finally reach their dreams. For months or years they concentrate all their energy on reaching a goal that they have set, continuing to strive toward it at every moment, never letting up for one moment. They are sure and certain that when they attain it, they will arrive at absolute happiness, at nirvana for all eternity. The closer they get to their goal, the stronger their desire becomes. It could be a question of someone in love who seeks the conquest of the man or woman who struck him or her like a bolt of lightning, a hard-to-get diploma that has suddenly been earned, or a fortune made after numerous efforts. But look at such people a mere five years later. The desire created by what they lacked has disappeared, the love stirred up by the one they were missing is no longer the same. Like lottery winners they no longer know what to do with their lives, how to give it meaning when they now have everything anyone could want. It becomes like a premature retreat where the universe shrinks a little more day after day. The whole paradox is there. You run after an ideal, and when you attain it the powerful motor of desire stops. The fuel of happiness is desire, which complicates things. For a happy person time passes quickly, very quickly. For a person who is bored, time passes very slowly. Philosopher Henri Bergson defined time as the uninterrupted welling up of unforeseen new things. This definition suggests a method for learning to be happy when you have succeeded in obtaining everything you wanted. Permanent movement is one of the keys to happiness. It means putting yourself in danger, knowing how to take risks, rediscovering what's missing in order to find new feelings. Change obliges us to continually adapt in order to create new equilibriums, in order to find new ways of being happy. It's important to learn how to always take on challenges and find new difficulties to overcome in order to feel better. The story never ends. The movement of life moves in step with the movement of happiness. Immobility destroys everything—intellectual functions, muscular potential, but also a talent for happiness.

Positive Psychology

This movement in psychology, born in the United States, has only recently arrived in France and risks overturning much conventional wisdom. For a long time psychology was harnessed to uncover, decode, and treat what went wrong in people. So things were based on the somewhat negative principle that the personality of an individual was first and foremost defined by trauma and neuroses. In the 1970s certain researchers, in contrast, thought that it would be interesting to emphasize the factors that contributed to a state of well-being and optimal functioning of the individual. In this perspective, positive psychology, born at the end of the 1990s, looks at the forces and values that animate a person, in all sectors of life—personal life, work, family, and spirituality. By improving your strengths and values, especially your strong points, you contribute to reinforcing your happiness.

Stop the Film in Order to Enjoy the Scene

It is essential that you know how to stop in order to better enjoy life. It's the opposite of one of those all-inclusive tours in which you absolutely must tick off each one of the tourist attractions without failing to take photos at every spot they point out to you so you can immortalize each and every moment. Once home you might say, "I was there and I saw everything." I think that in the end, watching a film on that country would have had about the same effect. The key is simply knowing how to stop the flow of time long enough that you enter into a resonance with the countryside, with a market scene, or with that fresh look from a child. Freeze the frame and think of each of your senses: hearing, smell, vision, taste, and touch. What information is being received? What exactly does it awaken in you? Concentrate on the most agreeable sensations and think only of them. Right there is where you are touching little moments of happiness and eternity. The important thing is not taking that photo that you can later show to others and file away, but instead it is to enjoy the immediate instant, the immediate force of the present moment. Procrastination is always putting off to tomorrow what could have been done that same day. There is also a procrastination of pleasure and of happiness. In your daily life don't forget to take regular breaks; stop on your way to work, smell the scents around you, linger with the smile of your child, and taste in-depth the flavors of a good meal shared with friends.

Stop Going over Negative Points

It has been shown that individuals who spend their time going over old, negative tales where they have been a victim or thinking about all there is that's wrong with their environment or in their professional life shorten their life spans. Turning in circles by ceaselessly thinking about what doesn't suit you wears out the body a little more day after day. Of course, you shouldn't act like an ostrich when you encounter a difficult situation, and you do need to analyze so that you understand better and can look for solutions so that things go more smoothly. In certain cases, after adequate reflection, you need also to know how to admit to yourself that there is no solution that will make the situation better. And once you do that it's useless to start once again going over the same problems. Some people have a tendency to wander around inside their brains, damaging their neurons and prodigiously annoying those around them. Did you know that in one study conducted on well-being in the workplace, colleagues who were whiners topped the list of discomforts? There is one good way to break this vicious circle. It consists of simply writing down on a piece of paper what's happening, opinions about it, the positions to take and not to take—once and for all. Then you put this piece of paper away, and you take it out and reread it every time you have a tendency to go around in circles about it again.

Working on Your Gross Domestic Happiness

The Kingdom of Bhutan is a little country in South Asia. It's a poor country that lives mainly on agriculture and tourism. But there is one thing that's special about it. In Bhutan the authorities have decided to talk not about gross domestic product, but about gross domestic happiness. Indicators of well-being are not material goods and the wealth of the inhabitants, but what makes them truly happy. On a personal level we could take inspiration from the philosophy of this country. The goal is not to be thinking about what we should do, but about what makes us truly happy. It's a difficult task that will lead to taking a second look at our lives, whether it has to do with leisure time; with those people with whom we share our most precious possession, our time; or what we buy, thinking we will please ourselves. We need to rethink everything in relation to our positive feelings. It's a question of sorting out what really makes us happy and what leaves us indifferent. Go over the week that just ended, choosing what you judge to be the best moments, those that in the end, you would like to relive as often as possible. Then think back on your various vacations, weekends, and meals shared with others and weigh them carefully. You will be surprised at the result. Happiness is not always where you thought it would be.

This exercise can be useful in making the choices we are confronted with day by day, in getting rid of situations where we find ourselves just wanting to do what everyone else is doing or getting stuck on the images of happy people that advertising projects. It's a good school for discovering the great power of saying *no,* for protecting oneself and not going along with just anything. In order not to lose the thread, I recommend that every day you select the best moment of the day and that you think hard about it so that it returns as often as possible. Also concentrate on what you shouldn't have done, the useless wasting of time, all those things you don't want to see repeated in the days and weeks ahead.

Accept Your Failures

Tal Ben-Shahar, who taught the practice of happiness at Harvard, highlights an important point—the right to make mistakes, the right not to be perfect and through this practice to achieve fullness. During his course he asked a student to draw a circle in chalk on the blackboard. The circle is drawn perfectly. He asked the student to remember how he drew at the age of two: pie shapes that were trying to look like circles. It's through having failed numerous times drawing circles in childhood that one day you get to a harmonious circle. You have to accept with serenity and without guilt that things don't work out right away. Understanding why things didn't work out is essential in order to move forward. When children are put under too much pressure, they can feel really demolished by an initial failure and risk falling into a cycle of failures if they feel crushed and above all if self-confidence is lost. It is of prime importance to look for a child's strong points that will act as footholds, as in rock climbing, providing the strength to move past the errors that are a normal part of learning. Perhaps one of the secrets of happiness lies hidden between the lines in childhood. We mustn't lose sight of the fact that by having the courage throughout our lives to make mistakes and to have things fail, we create a springboard for getting further and further ahead. It is essential to adopt good habits early on in order to be happy later. Developing positive thoughts is an important fuel for happiness. Look for the best in each present moment without always throwing yourself into the past or the future.

What Do Happy People Have More Of?

More than half of French people say they are happy or very happy; the results are similar in the United States. So for the other half who are still working on it, I would like to offer you a whole bundle of little tricks from happy people.

- External circumstances, including material success, is of little importance to them.
- They are aware that life is full of difficulties, and they integrate them into their cycle of existence.
- They are in harmony with themselves whether in their professional life, their love life, or their family or social life.
- They take care of their bodies and their minds as precious possessions.
- They don't seek continual approval in the eyes of others.
- They are in constant contact with their family, their friends, and their neighbors.
- They practice kindness, absence of judgment, and gratitude.
- They have a rich inner life: seeking deeper understanding, spirituality, religion.
- They know what they want, and they have a clearly defined life goal.
- And above all they live anchored firmly in the present without ruminating on and rehashing the past and without worrying or fantasizing about the future.

Avoid setting goals that are impossible to attain just so you can beat yourself up for not achieving them. Parents sometimes set goals for their children that correspond to what they would have liked to do themselves. They don't try to see the child and understand how she is different; instead they're thinking only of themselves. The child then is experienced by them as a means to their own social and narcissistic success, without regard for the child's true nature. There's nothing more terrible than spending our lives trying to achieve what doesn't suit us and that, moreover, is not within our grasp. Such a course of action is sowing the seeds for later depression, anxiety, and compensating behaviors such as excessive alcohol, obesity, smoking, and drugs. Happiness flows from the balance between who a person really is and the life he is living. The goal is to be yourself while pursuing the job you love regardless of what others think—and choosing the partner who really suits you, not the person who pleases those around you, your family, or your social contacts. You need to be in charge of your choices, without bad influences or bad reasons. This is the path to follow in order to love oneself and to love others, knowing how to receive, knowing how to give, and being fulfilled a little more every day in your job and in your relationships with others.

PRACTICING MEDITATION

In the deepest recesses of the human being, there are powerful means of self-healing that for the most part we are unaware of. The mind can act on the body in a spectacular way and can change things completely. Numerous scientific studies have shown that people who regularly practice meditation manage to reduce their blood pressure, slow their heart rate, and reduce their levels of stress. Other studies have demonstrated improved functioning of the immune system. On a neurological level researchers have discovered a significant improvement in intellectual and physical concentration in those who practice meditation daily. Certain results deserve to be promulgated—especially work that was presented at an international conference on cardiology in Orlando. Participants in this study practiced transcendental meditation for five years. Originating in India this is a technique of mental relaxation and consciousness development that is generally practiced in two twenty-minute sessions per day. It was observed that those who practiced meditation compared to those who didn't enjoyed a 43 percent decrease in death linked to cardiovascular disease. The study was carried out on 201 patients with an average age of fifty-nine. It is important to note that patients in both groups who were engaged in medical treatment continued those treatments. It is difficult to provide rational explanations for these results. Stress decreases sharply in those who practice meditation. The beginning of an explanation lies in the fact that stress is known to be a significant risk factor in cardiovascular disease.

The practice of meditation is within everyone's reach. All you need to do is to sit in silence, cross-legged on the ground with your gaze fixed on an object. Your eyes should be half closed, your arms resting on your thighs with the thumb and index finger forming a harmonious circle, the spine very straight. Sages of old compare this position to a stack of gold coins. In any case it is important not to be uncomfortable, which could disturb the proper unfolding of the meditation session. If need be don't hesitate to use a cushion to sit on or to sit in a chair if you have pain in the spine.

Once you have settled in, you need to learn to let go, to not think of anything except the object you're looking at. Very quickly, automatic thoughts appear, flashbacks about the near or distant past, thoughts about what you have to do in the coming days, weeks, or months. Becoming aware of these first parasitic thoughts and learning to let them fall away is an initial approach. You could compare this exercise to water that has been mixed with various impurities and stirred up. You just need to wait, without moving, for the impurities to settle onto the bottom, and the water will become clear and transparent. The object you choose to look at could be the point of a candle flame, for example. Learning how to concentrate all your energy and all your attention, even for only five minutes, on this shining tip will allow you to feel something strong and new in yourself. Imagine a laser ray spread over a whole wall. Nothing happens. But the same energy focused into a point can pierce the wall.

What counts in meditation is perseverance and regularity in the daily appointment with yourself. Breathing is essential. Learn to breathe calmly, slowly, and deeply by being aware that your own breathing makes it more possible to access the benefits of the meditation. There are many techniques and many books on this subject. I recommend first of all that you follow your instinct, finding out what works for you and, when you are ready, inventing your own method. Meditation is a fascinating trajectory to follow. It's a matter of finding the practice that is the best match to the inner you who wants to discover this path.

LITERATURE

Bunzeck, N., and E. Düzel. "Absolute coding of stimulus novelty in the human substantia nigra/VTA." *Neuron* 51(3) (2006): 369–79.

Ditzen, B., I. D. Neumann, G. Bodenmann, et al. "Effects of different kinds of couple interaction on cortisol and heart rate responses to stress in women." *Psychoneuroendocrinology* 32(5) (2007): 565–74.

Grewen K. M., S. S. Girdler, J. Amico, and K. C. Light. "Effects of partner support on resting oxytocin, cortisol, norepinephrine, and blood pressure before and after warm partner contact." *Psychosomatic Medicine* 67(4) (2005): 531–38.

Gruber, J., A. Kogan, J. Quoidbach, and I. B. Mauss. "Happiness is best kept stable: Positive emotion variability is associated with poorer psychological health." *Emotion* 13(1) (2013): 1–6.

Kraft, T. L., and S. D. Pressman. "Grin and bear it: The influence of manipulated facial expression on the stress response." *Psychological Science* 23(11) (2012): 1372–78.

Light, K. C., K. M. Grewen, and J. A. Amico. "More frequent partner hugs and higher oxytocin levels are linked to lower blood pressure and heart rate in premenopausal women." *Biological Psychology* 69(1) (2005): 5–21.

Massolt, E. T., P. M. van Haard, J. F. Rehfeld, et al. "Appetite suppression through smelling of dark chocolate correlates with changes in ghrelin in young women." *Regulatory Peptides* 161(1–3) (2010): 81–86.

McLauglin, N. "Happiness is a warm hug. Research suggests keeping employees happy is a great wellness program." *Modern Healthcare* 38(47) (2008): 18.

Paul-Labrador, M., D. Polk, J. H. Dwyer, et al. "Effects of a randomized controlled trial of transcendental meditation on components of the metabolic syndrome in subjects with coronary heart disease." *Archives of Internal Medicine* 166(11) (2006): 1218–24.

Tarnopolsky, M., J. D. Crane, D. I. Ogborn, et al. "Massage therapy attenuates inflammatory signaling after exercise-induced muscle damage." *Science Translational Medicine* 4(119) (2012): 119.

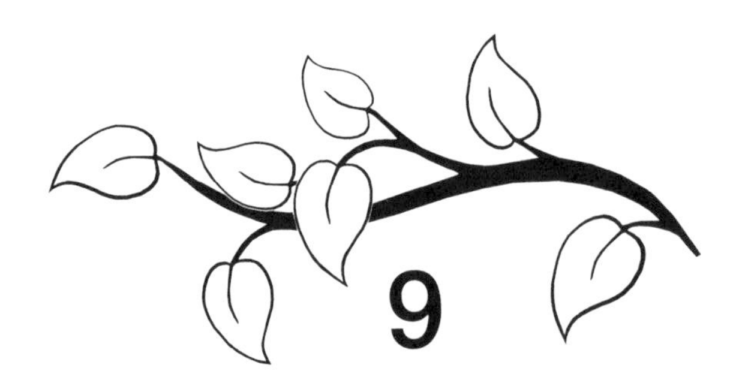

9

TRAINING YOUR BRAIN

My brain? That's my second favorite organ.

WOODY ALLEN

The brain only operates at 10 or 12 percent of its capacity. We're plunking away on a piano keyboard when we could be composing symphonies. The power of the brain is immense. The amount of gray matter is not—contrary to conventional wisdom—fixed in advance and does not diminish in quantity with time. We can push our intellectual capacities and our memory, a little like putting on the seven-league boots of folklore that enable the wearer to take giant steps so we can go faster and farther. We can act on ourselves and on others solely by the power of thought and concentration, sometimes reaching to the borders of mysterious worlds.

The brain contains 100 million neurons and, to the touch, has the consistency of a hard-boiled egg. Two of the basic fuels it uses are sugar and oxygen. The brain represents the most important function of the organism, yet very few people think much about preserving it, protecting it, and increasing its capacities. This is an essential point because the state of the brain determines the quality of life. It's all there in the brain: pleasure, enjoyment, intelligence. In caveman times it was muscular strength that created superiority and determined who controlled the territory. Today it's intelligence. Recent examples provided by the creators of Facebook, Google, and Microsoft show to what extent intelligence and imagination can build an empire from scratch. Improving cerebral performance means having a mind that is more alive and more responsive, with an increased memory capacity and more efficient functioning. The brain can be compared to muscles in the body. To have an athlete's body, it's not enough to work on the abdominals every day; you have to think of the other muscles too: the arms, the thighs, the legs. When it comes to the brain, it's the same thing. You need to exercise its various abilities every day to improve its performance. By working in this way, when something serious happens such as the appearance of a neurodegenerative disease (Alzheimer's, for example), the brain will be able to defer considerably the actual onset of the disease.

MODIFYING THE BRAIN'S STRUCTURE

Cognitive Reserves

As Michel Lejoyeux has said, "It's all those things that are changing that excite us, intrigue us, and stimulate us." It's true that a brain that is well muscled has an electric tool kit available that can limit the damage in case of a breakdown. This is called the cognitive reserve, which is a kind of reservoir of cerebral possibilities. In order to improve the cognitive reserve and reinforce the neuronal circuits, you need to exercise daily. For example, if you push yourself to try to understand a scientific train of thought when you don't have that training, the process will stimulate new areas of your brain. In the same way doing two things at once (phoning and reading a newspaper) calls upon new circuits in the brain. Throwing yourself into a cooking recipe when all you know how to do is boil noodles is another example of the same activation. Contrary to popular wisdom new neurons can be formed every day, regardless of your age. This concept can surprise people who think that we are born with a predetermined supply of neurons that dwindles as the years go by. Not at all. The future of your brain is in your hands.

It will become what you make of it. The choice is yours; either let it decline over the years or pursue daily training so that its performance continually improves. However, having a fast and super powerful hard drive of brain capacity requires setting up a real program of overall personal health. Your brain reserves are in direct relationship with having a healthy lifestyle; your cognitive reserves are linked to external stimulation; and psychological and affective reserves are connected directly to your social relationships.

Having better cerebral reserves means bestowing on yourself the ability to considerably delay the onset of neurodegenerative disease by increasing the number of synaptic connections while at the same time optimizing the ability to recruit new neuronal circuits. The brain then becomes more flexible and is more resistant to disease. The formation of these alternative neural networks is like building a dike against the kind of pathologies that damage cerebral tissue. We need to improve our storage space, our transmission bandwidth for information, and also stimulate our capacity for imagination—which we can do by remembering the Victor Hugo quotation: "Imagination is intelligence being erected."

Watching over Your General State

It's clear that the general state of the body directly impacts the state of the brain. The brain needs oxygen in order to function properly. The oxygen is carried by hemoglobin in the blood moving through the arteries. If the arteries narrow because the plaque caused by atherosclerosis is gradually clogging them, the brain will be poorly irrigated, and worst case, a completely blocked artery will lead to a stroke with horrible damage such as hemiplegia, or loss of vision or language. It is important, therefore, to take care that the arteries do not get blocked so that the essential fuel the brain needs arrives properly in its cells.

Cholesterol needs to be monitored regularly since, when it's too high, it participates in the formation of plaque that gets deposited in the arteries (see chapter 2). It can be lowered with a diet that is low in cholesterol or, if that is not sufficient, by medication prescribed by your doctor. You can also help your condition by using industrial food products such as yogurts and margarines that contain phytosterols that are capable of lowering the cholesterol level in the blood by 10 to 15 percent. In addition, we need to monitor other fats in the blood such as the triglycerides.

Diabetes is also implicated in the formation of plaque (see chapter 2). In fact, there are significant links between diabetes and the incidence of strokes. Whether it's a diabetes that is being treated with insulin or type 2 diabetes in older people that is treated with medication, it is important to never allow an excess level of sugar in the blood. Excess sugar acts as a poison and damages all the blood passageways, whether it be those involving the heart with a myocardial infarction (heart attack), the vessels of the legs with arteritis, or the eyes.

Finally, high blood pressure is a real scourge because it can go on for years without causing symptoms, which could be, for example, headaches or an impression of flies moving in front of your eyes. In certain cases the pressure is normal when resting and excessively elevated at certain times of day. There is a simple way to clear up this question. All you need to do is have your doctor install a little unit on your belt for twenty-four hours to record the arterial pressure at regular intervals. This procedure will allow your practitioner to see if the arterial pressure during the day always stays within normal limits. High blood pressure also impacts the small vessels in the eyes. These exceedingly fine vessels are very sensitive to elevated arterial pressure. The examination of the back of the eye done by ophthalmologists can determine that these little vessels are not suffering and remain undamaged. High blood pressure can insidiously creep in over the course of the years, causing very severe damage to the organism. The brain is one of the first areas to suffer the consequences. Such damage is all the more regrettable since all the therapeutic means necessary for treating and stabilizing arterial pressure do exist today. Just as families have a thermometer for taking one's temperature, it would also be useful to have a home blood pressure monitor. It is clear that the discovery of high blood pressure ought to systematically lead to a complete medical exam that will investigate, on the one hand, the possible causes of the hypertension and that will, on the other hand, evaluate the damage that may already have been done.

Learning and Thinking

Repeated thoughts can succeed in modifying the structure of your brain. Scientists at Harvard University asked an initial group of subjects to play a regular sequence of piano notes with their right and left hands starting with the thumb, going up to the pinky and back—*do re mi fa so fa mi re do* and so on—for a lengthy session every day for five days. At the end of five days, they observed on MRIs a modification in the area of the brain corresponding to finger movement that had grown in size in comparison to the MRIs taken before the exercises. A second group of subjects was asked not to play the piano notes but to be sitting beside the pianist at each session and mentally imagine that they were performing the same exercise on the piano. The surprise was that the MRIs of the nonplayers showed the same modifications in the brain as those who played. Through concentration, imagination, and thought, the spectators came up with the same results as the actors. Through the learning of specific movements, thoughts, or reasoning, the brain can, day after day, beef up and become stronger. Similarly, if you teach people to juggle every day, the areas of the brain that correspond to the ability to juggle are going to develop. An MRI can show the brain grow in the corresponding areas. Conversely, if the person stops juggling, the areas that have increased in volume will return to a smaller size several months later.

By comparing the brains of twins who were identical at birth, it can be seen that a few years later they are no longer the same at all because of the experiences they have undergone and their learning in various domains. Thanks to progress in cerebral imaging, the ability to study the brain online allows us to understand the point to which our thoughts and our actions alter the very structure of the brain. What is marvelous is that although the brain is contained in the limited space of the cranium, it always knows how to make room by folding into convolutions. Imagine that you're putting a sheet away in a box—it will end up in numerous folds in order to fit. This is exactly what happens with your brain inside the skull. Specialists have shown that if you were to unfold the brain on the surface of a table, it would take up two square meters (2 square yards) with a thickness of 3 millimeters (0.1 inches). The brain has a true plasticity, which means it is able to change, evolve permanently, and grow in the activated regions or reduce in size in areas that fall asleep. People who find themselves profoundly changed because of a new calling, various sensations, or new learning will see that the corresponding areas of the brain modify on an MRI. Conversely, if we are always repeating the same actions, if our thoughts are always turning in circles, the brain will only be working to a limited capacity. The brain is idling when it is just reproducing repetitive activities, like Charlie Chaplin in the movie *Modern Times.* It's as if the brain has been put on standby. We need to teach people of all ages to do things they couldn't do before in order to stimulate areas of the brain that have fallen asleep and are asking no more than to be kept alive.

REGENERATE YOUR BRAIN

Break the Routine

In the deepest part of the brain, there is a small, secret area called the hippocampus that actually works like radar for new facts. When something new appears the hippocampus compares the incoming information to what is already stored. If the new material is confirmed, the hippocampus will send signals to other areas of the brain so that they produce dopamine, the pleasure hormone. Research has shown that what is new stimulates memory.

The brain has the capacity to wake up and increase its power when it is not subjected to routine. Habits and repetition constitute a destructive poison for intellectual abilities. Rapidity of thought, memory, and intelligence need change as an essential fuel so that they remain reliable, in high performance mode, and do not unavoidably deteriorate over the course of time. Neurodegenerative diseases are a real scourge and continue to increase. How many people as they grow old undergo an alteration in intellectual function and consider the ankylosis, or rigor, of their brains to be inevitable? That is the moment when they do precisely the opposite of what they should do to remain in good health; they put themselves into routine and repetitive circuits as if to protect themselves. And it is precisely in this attempt at protecting themselves that they put themselves in danger. The absence of small, daily dangers, daily tasks that are too easy, and the lack of things unforeseen and new social contacts constitute the real risks. Present-day society gums up our efforts: the escalator, the automobile, softer and softer food—everything is designed to diminish physical exercise and also intellectual effort. Given the same age the mortality rate of retired people is higher than people who stay engaged. Activities like golf, bridge, or crossword puzzles are not enough to produce beneficial effects on your health. The brain is not fooled by what looks like distractions for children disguised as pseudoactivities for seniors.

Numerous studies have been conducted on rats in order to better understand the impact of routine or change on this animal. By comparing caged rats, some of them subjected to frequent change and others to a fixed routine running like clockwork, the researchers very quickly noticed that changes appeared. The routine group showed, in comparison to the other group, a decrease in libido and in appetite, and they moved around very little in their cages, curling up for whole days at a time in a corner. Another study, also with rats, conducted by Professor Michael Bardo of the psychology department at the University of Kentucky, showed that things that were perceived as surprising provoked the same effects as cocaine in the brains of the rodents. These results allow us to understand why people on vacation sometimes feel a little more tired or even more depressed than usual. We agree with the goal of vacations for feeling good, having fun, and enjoying well-being—but vacations that are full of repetition and have no change reduce the production of pleasure hormones. Vacation homes or cottages, for many people, definitely mean the absence of change and adventure and amount to substituting one routine for another. The official criteria for well-being, relaxation, and leisure time are unfortunately stereotyped.

We need to dare to break conventions and redefine what really pleases us by moving outside how others see us. If you like doing housework, dare to think and say that you do; if you adore scrubbing or sanding a hardwood floor, don't talk about it like a chore but as a time of pleasure and relaxation. The beginning of happiness is to dare to love what others hate. We need to move outside conventions when need be. It's the opposite of what we learn in school where we have to always fit the mold. Our education authorities ought to institute courses for learning adaptability and moving outside the beaten path. It is there that the real keys to success are to be found. Humans are like serpents—those who don't manage to change their skins at the right moment die little by little.

SELF-CONTROL

The Willpower Circuit

We have all been confronted with the gap that exists between what we plan to do, the objectives that we set ourselves, and reality. All too often good resolutions don't pan out and we find ourselves in situations of chronic failure that erode our self-image. When this happens people feel weak and stew about their lack of willpower. The most common charade in attempting to get out of that is to put off to tomorrow what we planned to do today but that didn't work out. However, tomorrow shows up and is very much like the day before with the same failures . . . and years pass with nothing ever getting done. The best example of these failures arising from a chronic lack of self-control is illustrated by diets for losing weight. More than half the population wants to lose weight, and yet it's an unprecedented fiasco. Of those who follow a diet, no matter which one, 95 percent put the weight back on during the following year. At the same time I have always been upset by the level of dietary knowledge in patients who come to consult me about losing weight. They have a deep knowledge of the subject—which foods to eliminate and which to consume—and they know that there is no medication that is not dangerous in the treatment of obesity. Added to that is, generally speaking, a solid experience of the ineffective methods that are on the market. I often have the impression that I'm speaking to experts in nutrition for whom I can do nothing . . . or almost nothing.

The Marshmallow Experiment

In the 1970s an experiment was conducted on four-year-old children, and it's only today that we have the complete results. Scientists working under Stanford University professor Walter Mischel placed children, one by one, in front of two plates. One plate contained one marshmallow, the other two marshmallows. The researcher made clear to each child that he was going to leave the room. If the children succeeded in waiting without pressing a buzzer placed on the table to call the researcher back, they would get to eat two marshmallows. If they didn't have the patience to wait, they would only get one. A hidden camera in the room facilitated the observation of the behavior of each one of the children. Certain of them adopted various strategies to hold out, and others wolfed down the sweets without waiting. Forty years later the scientists looked into what had become of the children and compared the data to the results of the earlier tests. It seems that the children who had no trouble resisting without pushing the buzzer had life paths that were different from the other group. Overall, they had done better in university competitions, had better careers, and enjoyed a higher standard of living. They lived in happier households and were in better health. Here we have an interesting educational model using, through clever strategies of the brain, the springboard of willpower to confront obstacles in life and move forward.

The common denominator among all these individuals is that they don't manage to hold up over the long term—they end up cracking, and their lack of willpower makes them sad. I think that if you want to achieve good, lasting results in losing weight, you have to begin with the most essential thing: self-control. It's not just a word—it's one of the keys for transforming daily defeat into success. In fact, self-control works on you and reinforces itself, just as working on your muscles creates hard abdominals. Achieving a proper balance between principles of reason, temptations, and pleasure depends entirely on the brain, which has an essential role to play in the control of impulses.

Recent scientific discoveries have shown that willpower is directly related to the state of the brain. Will and self-control are dependent on the energy that the brain has available. In practice, if you wear yourself out with difficult tasks, less energy remains to resist. The principle is to know how to concentrate your energy and not squander it. Making good use of our energy—using it for what's essential—is crucial in optimizing self-control. The quantity of cerebral energy we have available is not infinite—it gets used up quickly and we need to make choices if we want our desires to be realized.

No doubt you have experienced the following situation: right in the middle of a weight-loss diet, you find yourself at a dinner where the atmosphere is especially tense either for professional reasons or because of interpersonal conflict. Some part of your energy is going to be focused on resolving these tensions. Suddenly, there's not much left to control your eating. You're on the verge of cracking and tucking into dishes that aren't worth it. It's exactly at such a moment that you will hate yourself for your lack of willpower. The solution however is easy; drop the personal conflicts and concentrate only on controlling your food intake. You also need to remember that having alcoholic beverages lowers your defense system and decreases your self-control.

Exercises in Self-Control

Self-control requires a certain number of exercises to bolster it. Here are a few keys for a day-by-day training program just as in a physical education course.

- The wave principle: Think hard about a wave that rises up and up, getting larger and larger, and then crashing onto the beach. Mentally compare this wave to something you want, such as for example a pastry you want to gobble down or a cigarette that is just waiting for your lighter. Several waves later, your desire will disappear naturally.
- Avoid risky situations: It's clear that in order not to burn up too quickly the amount of willpower available in the brain, you need to avoid risky situations that will require too much energy to resolve. Shopping in the deli just before lunch hour requires a lot of cerebral fuel spent on resisting. After such a battle you won't have enough energy of resistance left to resolve the next conflicts.
- Live in the present moment and don't put things off to tomorrow: In order to avoid unpleasant situations that you're only going to regret, you need to fully experience the present moment, based on the key point that what does not get done today will never get done. In order to build self-control and increase the field of one's own willpower, you need to acquire the means to do so. They are not innate and need to be worked on every day. Living fully in the present and not in the past or the future constitutes the first stage. Here's an example: You have resolved a few days ago that you would lose weight, and yet there you go beginning your day with a croissant whose aroma attracted you. As you know it takes seven kilometers (four miles) of jogging to burn off the calories in a croissant. It would be a mistake to tell yourself that given where you're at, the diet can wait until tomorrow. The excess is going to accumulate so much that each day it will become more difficult to attain the goals that you have set yourself. On the contrary, you need to correct your aim immediately, just as when sailing

you trim your sail looking for that new wind that will move you forward.

The rise in strength of our inner force in order to have better self-control constitutes the energy and is the essential motor for succeeding in attaining the goals we set ourselves. It's a real training that we need to force ourselves to follow on a daily basis. Lack of self-control provokes a continual backsliding in the personality and will one day create a big gap between what people really are and their daily life. When the gap widens it opens the door to various systems of compensation for the resulting misfortune—excessive consumption of alcohol leading to alcoholism, a flood of calories leading to obesity, smoking or drugs, antidepressants—all trying to keep you afloat in a mess that never ends.

How You Move Affects Your Brain

There are certain movements that can condition the mind and provoke reflexes in thinking. The kinds of movement you make on a daily basis are important for training yourself to activate your inner strength. Here are a few examples.

- Like a dancer train yourself to hold yourself upright and not be hunched. When walking imagine that you have a pile of books balanced on the top of your head. The effect is immediate; by carrying yourself better you will feel better able to stand up to others and to situations and also more able to be in control of yourself.
- Use the same approach in sitting—by flexing your legs rather than bending.
- Try as much as possible during the day to use your left hand (if you are right-handed)—when you pick up a cup of coffee or when you press the elevator button for example. This change stimulates cerebral circuits that are habitually asleep and activates a new energy for optimizing self-control using the simple gestures of everyday life.

BOOST YOUR MEMORY

The Importance of Memory

The performance of our memory ability is essential. Early on we learn to what an extent this function is fundamental. An excellent memory allows us to be successful in scholarly exams and university competitions. During my study of medicine, I was very quickly confronted with the strength of memory that had to be developed in order to make it through difficult times. In later life seniors are haunted by the fear of losing their memory along with the specter of Alzheimer's lurking in the background (see text box below). We now understand that the more individuals use brain functions and increase memory performance, the more they will be protected against Alzheimer's. The appearance of the disease cannot be prevented, but it will happen much later in life, which changes everything; the story is not the same for an illness that begins at seventy compared to one that begins at eighty-five.

Alzheimer's Disease

Alzheimer's disease is a fearful degenerative pathology that affects one man in eight and one women in four. It is not an illness that is linked to aging since young individuals can be struck by it. What is terrifying about it is that its victims progressively lose their memory, their identity, and their language. They no longer recognize those close to them, they become strangers to themselves, and they even lose any reason for living. Once the illness has taken hold, there are no medications to stop the irreversible destruction of nerve cells and the patients die after a few years of real torture. Up to now we have not found the cause of this pathology. However, there are several risk factors including cholesterol, diabetes, high blood pressure, smoking, and obesity. The link is easy to understand because if arteries that are intended to irrigate the brain become clogged with atherosclerosis, proper cerebral function will be compromised.

Besides these known factors there are other factors that can change how things turn out. Physical and intellectual activity constitutes a formidable rampart for protecting yourself against this disease. One initial statistic speaks volumes: one half hour of uninterrupted physical exercise per day reduces the risk of developing Alzheimer's during one's lifetime by 40 percent. It's simple and it works really well. The other side of protection is training your mind every day to increase its performance. When you realize that in a vacation of three weeks you lose twenty points on your IQ, you can imagine the risk of retirement.

Stepping Up Performance

Short-term memory is stimulated when, for example, a friend tells you his telephone number out loud. You have no way to write it down, and you absolutely must remember it. Short-term memory can retain about seven elements for twenty seconds. If the telephone number is (061) 253-8609, a standard ten digits, it is much easier to remember it as: 061 253 860, which is only three elements. For the final digit you could think of it as the last thing before nothing. The association of ideas is another way of improving mental performance. Repeating these little exercises gradually builds up your memory and improves its performance. You can also start learning a foreign language in order to stimulate the memorization capacity of your neurons. Sometimes you can help yourself remember by connecting blocks of numbers to external facts in order to anchor them more firmly in your memory. For example, if you have to remember the numbers 1, 4, 9, 2, it is easier to remember 1492 and connect it to the date that Christopher Columbus discovered America.

There are numerous simple and practical exercises for bringing a dynamism to your memory. Some of them help you save time such as learning your Social Security number by heart or your passport number if you travel a lot. Memorizing your Social Security number will help you fill out forms more quickly. Each time you reactivate these numbers, you are stimulating your memory and surprising those around you who, unlike you, have to go fumbling through papers to find the right number. You can also help yourself with simple mnemonic techniques such as connecting a department name to an anniversary date or an address. Associating ideas together is an excellent way to activate the meninges. A useful little exercise is to repeat to oneself new information, such as an unknown word from a foreign language, just before falling asleep and to memorize at the end of each week the new words that have been learned.

Eat Fish—It's Scientific!

Eating fish makes you smarter, and it's good for your memory. Sometimes there can be truth in popular sayings. In fact, the accuracy of this saying has recently been discovered. In 2011 a team of scientists presented an astonishing scientific study to the prestigious annual meeting of the Radiological Society of North America in Chicago. Dr. Cyrus Raji studied a group of 260 adults for ten years. He divided them into two groups. The first group ate fish several times a week, and the second never ate fish at all. The results showed that in those who ate fish between one and four times a week, there was maintenance activity going on during the ten years that affected the gray matter in the brain in several cerebral regions and especially in one key area, the hippocampus, which plays a key role in memory. Usually, the gray matter and the hippocampus gradually shrink in volume over the course of the years, but definitely not in those who eat fish.

Since we do not currently have available any effective medications for protecting and stimulating memory, this discovery is essential. By comparing the volume of gray matter in the two groups of patients, the researchers established that the risk of developing minor memory problems or Alzheimer's disease in the next five years was reduced to one-fifth. The doctors also realized that by having both groups of patients take memory tests after ten years of study, those patients who ate fish had much better memories and they also scored higher on all their cognitive tests.

Warning—Danger!

Certain fish, such as eel, absolutely must be avoided. The problem with eel is that it concentrates environmental toxins (dioxin, PCBs, and methylmercury, but also heavy metals such as lead, cadmium, and mercury) and has no way of breaking them down. When we eat eel the toxins from its organism move into ours, and they have a tendency to become lodged in organs that are rich in lipids such as the gray matter of the brain. Other fish, such as carp, barbel, bream, and silurid, although they are less contaminated by PCBs, should also be eaten as seldom as possible. These river fish are victims of contamination and can in turn contaminate us.

The other surprising discovery of this team is the discovery of the importance of the cooking method: depending on how you cook the fish, you will benefit or not from its protective effects on your memory. In fact, fish that is grilled, steamed, baked, or wrapped in foil or parchment has positive effects on memory while fish that is deep fried loses its protective character. These differences are explained by the fact that the component in fish that acts on memory is called omega-3. The omega-3s are good fats known for a long time for their beneficial effects on the cardiovascular system. This is supported by the fact that the Japanese and the Inuit, being great consumers of fish, have a very low incidence of heart attacks. The omega-3 fats act by reducing the quantity of certain harmful fats that are circulating in the blood such as the triglycerides, and in so doing they make the blood flow better. What is new is their effect on the brain. The sensitivity of omega-3 fats to temperature requires a gentle cooking of the fish in order to maximize their benefits for your health.

In practice, fish with a low level of omega-3s are as follows: pollock, coalfish, cod, whiting, sole, ling, skate, hake, burbot or monkfish, plaice, and dab. Fish with a medium level of omega-3s are as follows: red mullet (red gurnard or surmullet), anchovy, sea bass, sea bream, turbot, pike, and halibut. Lastly, fish that are rich in omega-3s are as follows: salmon, tuna, sardine, mackerel, and herring. Not only do all these fish contain omega-3s—they also are rich in protein, minerals such phosphorus, and trace elements such as iodine, zinc, copper, selenium, and fluorine not to mention vitamins A, D, and E. From a health point of view, it is beneficial to eat fish that are both rich in omega-3s and, at the same time, those least contaminated by toxins.

LITERATURE

Abel, E. L., and M. L. Kruger. "Age heterogamy and longevity: Evidence from Jewish and Christian cemeteries." *Biodemography and Social Biology* 54(1) (2008): 1–7.

Abel, E. L., and M. L. Kruger. "Symbolic significance of initials on longevity." *Perceptual and Motor Skills* 104(1) (2007): 179–82.

Abel, E. L., M. M. Kruger, and K. Pandya. "Sopranos but not tenors live longer." *Aging Male* 15(2) (2012): 109–10.

Almqvist, C., F. Garden, A. S. Kemp, et al. "Effects of early cat or dog ownership on sensitisation and asthma in a high-risk cohort without disease-related modification of exposure." *Paediatric and Perinatal Epidemiology* 24(2) (2010): 171–78.

Bardo, M. T., R. L. Donohew, and N. G. Harrington. "Psychobiology of novelty seeking and drug seeking behavior." *Behavioural Brain Research* 77(1–2) (1996): 23–43.

Bedrosian, T. A., L. K. Fonken, J. C. Walton, et al. "Dim light at night provokes depression-like behaviors and reduces CA1 dendritic spine density in female hamsters." *Psychoneuroendocrinology* 36(7) (2011): 1062–69.

Bjørnerem, A., L. A. Ahmed, L. Jørgensen, et al. "Breast-feeding protects against hip fracture in postmenopausal women: The Tromsø study." *Journal of Bone and Mineral Research* 26(12) (2011): 2843–50.

Brock, K. E., G. Berry, L. A. Brinton, et al. "Sexual, reproductive and contraceptive risk factors for carcinoma-in-situ of the uterine cervix in Sydney." *Medical Journal of Australia* 150(3) (1989): 125–30.

Choi, K. S. "The effects of teacher expectancy and self-expectancy on performance." *Shinrigaku Kenkyu* 58(3) (1987): 181–85; article in Japanese.

Cutt, H., B. Giles-Corti, M. Knuiman, and V. Burke. "Dog ownership, health and physical activity: A critical review of the literature." *Health Place* 13(1) (2007): 261–72.

Freudenheim, J. L., J. R. Marshall, J. E. Vena, et al. "Lactation history and breast cancer risk." *American Journal of Epidemiology* 146(11) (1997): 932–38.

Ganzer, C., and C. Zauderer. "Promoting a brain-healthy lifestyle." *Nursing Older People* 23(7) (2011): 24–27.

Ho, A. J., C. A. Raji, P. Saharan, et al. "Hippocampal volume is related to body mass index in Alzheimer's disease." *Neuroreport* 22(1) (2011): 10–14.

Kaur, B., E. A. Chiocca, and T. P. Cripe. "Oncolytic HSV-1 virotherapy: Clinical experience and opportunities for progress." *Current Pharmaceutical Biotechnology* 13(9) (2012): 1842–51.

Kraft, T. L., and S. D. Pressman. "Grin and bear it: The influence of manipulated facial expression on the stress response." *Psychological Science* 23(11) (2012): 1372–78.

Mischel, W., E. B. Ebbeson, and A. R. Zeiss. "Cognitive and attentional mechanisms in delay of gratification." *Journal of Personality and Social Psychology* 21(2) (1972): 204–18.

Pace, T. W., L. T. Negi, D. D. Adame, et al. "Effect of compassion meditation on neuroendocrine, innate immune and behavioral responses to psychosocial stress." *Psychoneuroendocrinology* 34(1) (2009): 87–98.

Paul-Labrador, M., D. Polk, J. H. Dwyer, et al. "Effects of a randomized controlled trial of transcendental meditation on components of the metabolic syndrome in subjects with coronary heart disease." *Archives of Internal Medicine* 166(11) (2006): 1218–24.

Presl, J. "Pregnancy and breast feeding decreases the risk of ovarian carcinoma." *Ceskoslovenská Gynekologie* 46(7) (1981): 541–44; article in Czech.

Radon, K., A. Schulze, and D. Nowak. "Inverse association between farm animal contact and respiratory allergies in adulthood: Protection, underreporting or selection?" *Allergy* 61(4) (2006): 443–46.

Rainforth, M. V., R. H. Schneider, S. I. Nidich, et al. "Stress reduction programs in patients with elevated blood pressure: A systematic review and meta-analysis." *Current Hypertension Reports* 9(6) (2007): 520–28.

Raji. C. A., K. I. Erickson, O. L. Lopez, et al. "Regular fish consumption and age-related brain gray matter loss." *American Journal of Preventive Medicine* 47(4) (2014): 444–51.

Schneider, R., S. Nidich, J. M. Kotchen, et al. "Abstract 1177: Effects of stress reduction on clinical events in African Americans with coronary heart disease; A randomized controlled trial." *Circulation* 120 (2009): S461.

Schneider, R. H., K. G. Walton, J. W. Salerno, and S. I. Nidich. "Cardiovascular disease prevention and health promotion with the transcendental meditation program and Maharishi consciousness-based health care." *Ethnicity & Disease* 16(3 suppl. 4) (2006): 15–26.

Weinstein, R. S., H. H. Marshall, L. Sharp, and M. Botkin. "Pygmalion and the student: Age and classroom differences in children's awareness of teacher expectations." *Child Development* 58(4) (1987): 1079–93.

Xu, X., A. Aron, L. Brown, et al. "Reward and motivation systems: A brain mapping study of early-stage intense romantic love in Chinese participants." *Human Brain Mapping* 32(2) (2011): 249–57.

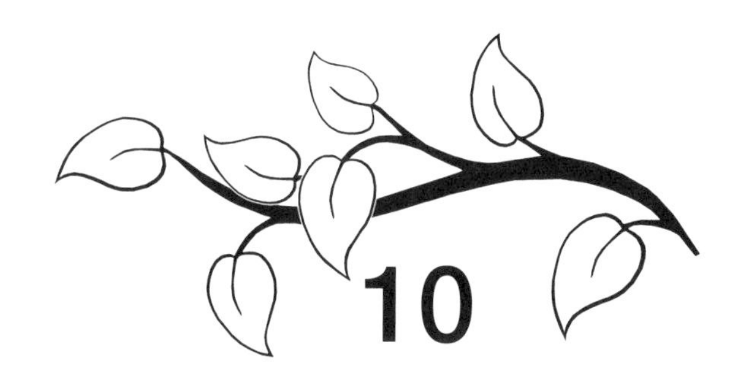

10

MAGNETISM, CLAIRVOYANCE, AND MYSTERIOUS HEALING

Looking all very natural, the supernatural is around us everywhere.

Jules Supervielle

What if we had close to science-fiction powers, forces available that we didn't even suspect existed? Myth or reality? Are these powers reserved for a minority of individuals, or can we all learn how to develop them? Incredible scientific progress today is allowing us to uncover limits that are difficult to imagine, limits that push the boundaries of the normal. Often in medicine when we can't make a diagnosis in defining a patient's disorder, we say it's "in her head," which is a very handy catchall expression to cover up what we don't understand. For example, patients who suffered from a gastric ulcer were for many years assigned to the category of those suffering from psychiatric illness—until the day came when we realized that the ulcer was caused by a bacteria that could be eliminated by a simple antibiotic treatment. A great many paranormal phenomena are systematically grouped with manifestations related to the psychic. But perhaps there is a hidden dimension that is not apparent at first glance: déjà vu (literally "already seen") experiences, telepathy, clairvoyance that allows knowing in advance what will happen, and spontaneous healings are prime examples. If science were to seriously take a close look at these phenomena, what would really be brought to light?

SCIENTIFIC STUDIES THAT STIR THINGS UP

In order to understand these phenomena that some people call paranormal, a certain number of scientific and medical experiments were conducted following rigorous methodologies.

Déjà Vu Experiences: A Powerful Tool for Enhancing Your Memory

What characterizes déjà vu experiences is the mixture of simultaneous familiarity, newness, and strangeness—without being able to connect what is happening to anything in the past. International teams have explored this phenomenon, in particular Dr. Adachi in Japan. Several elements have emerged. First of all, the impressions of déjà vu occurred most often with individuals who were young and had a high level of education. No differences were found relating to sex, place of residence, or lifestyle. The second point that emerged is that the more the person benefited from high performance memory, the higher the probability that the person would have episodes of déjà vu. These findings raise a paradoxical point: the person, in searching through the far reaches of memory, does not manage to find any reason for the déjà vu and ends up concluding that memory is failing. What is happening is precisely the opposite since this person is benefiting from high-performance mnemonic functions. In fact, at some moments, the brain begins to function like a high-speed computer without our being aware of it. The flash that happens corresponds to analogous situations experienced in the past that have not completely risen to the surface. Let's take an example. You arrive in a country you've never visited before. At a street corner you decide to stop for refreshments in a café. You order a soda, and at that precise moment you have the distinct impression of having already experienced exactly this scene in this same café. You search through your memories, but nothing appears. You're like a detective chasing clues. At a nearby table a woman is wearing a summer dress with a pattern of pink flowers. At no moment do you notice that, however. And yet, during your childhood you saw your mother wearing the same pattern. This detail is enough to give the impression of déjà vu to the scene. There are other interpretations of déjà vu. For Sigmund Freud déjà vu was *déjà rêvé,* or already dreamed. Imagine that you dreamed of a situation and you forgot about it when you awoke. Some years later this situation repeats but you are unable to dredge up the slightest link to the forgotten dream.

Recent research has made clear that contrary to popular wisdom, paying attention will not necessarily help someone to see better. In practice, researchers have shown that visual data can reach our consciousness independently of the attention we direct toward it. This means that we can manage to see without seeing—that is, memorize visual elements without being aware at the time that that's what we've been doing. This particularity allows us to explain certain déjà vu phenomena. Our memory is a structure that is in constant evolution.

When we think of our memories, imperceptibly, without intending to, we transform them ever so slightly each time. This is how, over the course of some years, false memories appear. They have never existed, although the person is convinced otherwise. Scientific teams have studied the impact of advertising that fabricates false memories. Tests have shown that consumers who have seen TV commercials carefully describing the pleasure of tasting some sweet product are convinced that a few weeks earlier they tried that dessert when in fact they have never tasted it.

TELEPATHY UNDER THE SCANNER

Telepathy is a fascinating thing in an era of cell phones, texting, and e-mail. Being able to communicate with someone on the other side of the planet—being able to influence his thoughts simply by concentrating might make your head spin. But what is really going on?

A Mysterious Phenomenon

There are many experiments on telepathy that can't always be explained. This is the case with a study conducted by Dr. Rudolph Peters at Cambridge University in England. It all began when this scientist met with a mother whose son suffered from intellectual disability. Besides his disability the boy also had very limited eyesight. The ophthalmologist was very surprised to find that contrary to what he was expecting, the visual abilities of the young boy were perfect. He then decided to try an experiment. He had the mother leave the room where the child was. The boy's vision fell apart completely. He did the tests over again, and each time he found that the child could succeed on the tests only if his mother was in the same room. He formed the hypothesis that there could be small, imperceptible signs agreed upon beforehand between the mother and the child, without the scientist being able to perceive them. Without warning the child he did the tests over again but with the mother hidden in a nearby room. The visual tests were a success. They went further with the experiment. At a distance of eight kilometers (five miles) from the laboratory, they showed the mother, in random order, a series of cards containing letters and numbers. Over the telephone the doctor asked the boy what number or letter was shown. Whereas statistically he should have been able to provide the right answer in 10 percent of the cases at best, the different trials with the boy and his mother provided the right answer in 32 percent of the cases. This is not an isolated observation. We would need to reproduce this experiment on a larger scale to be able to verify the data.

Often people feel that someone is going to call them or that they're going to receive a text or e-mail, and precisely what they intuited happens. It is interesting to note that experiences of telepathy generally involve people who knew each other beforehand. Telepathy between people who don't know each other is more rare.

Telepathy and E-mail

Biologist Rupert Sheldrake wanted to test the possibility of communication by telepathy in relation to e-mail. To do so he chose four individuals to send e-mails. The participants had to guess, one minute before the sending took place which of the four persons was going to send the e-mail. After 552 trials 43 percent succeeded in choosing the right person, which is very much higher than standard probability—around 25 percent. It is impossible to this day to find an explanation for this phenomenon. It would be necessary to reproduce such experiments with larger numbers of participants in order to have a better interpretation of the data.

The Beginnings of an Explanation?

There are a few scraps of explanation regarding the phenomenon of telepathy. Think of some popular expressions that refer to two people: "You could see a current connecting them" or "I feel something from that person—I feel drawn to her" or "I feel no connection with him." In order to try to understand these feelings of attraction and repulsion between people, a great many scientific studies have been conducted in the last few decades. Certain elements have been identified that allow us to better analyze what is taking place beyond the social or psychological context. It is true that the attraction between a man and a woman can, in the end, be the result of the action of a family, societal, or advertising model. In unconscious ways we can integrate models of what we take to be the ideal spouse into our subconscious. The model may turn out to be a young film star, the hero of some novel, the ideal son-in-law that the parents are suggesting, or the model may range from the head of the class to the rebellious dunce.

Any model is possible—in harmony with or in opposition to what the external world proposes. Certain people find serenity in choosing the ideal son-in-law or the perfect daughter-in-law, in order to continue to feel loved by their parents. Others, conversely, project themselves onto opposing models so they can have the feeling of affirming themselves and living intensely by breaking from an obligation that was imposed on them and not agreed to. In both cases the result risks being the same: a choice made to please or out of a reaction that does not necessarily correspond to one's deepest wish. Outside the psychological dimension of the choice of a partner, numerous studies have explored other traits. It seems that attraction is more intense in cases of significant genetic differences and that the sense of smell plays a not insignificant role in sexual desire toward the other person. Odor plays a part as a sexual stimulus, in particular odor from the armpits and from pubic hair for example.

There are still unexplained dimensions in attraction and communication between humans . . . but not only between humans.

Other scientific studies have been conducted on the transmission of thoughts between animals and humans. For example, many cases have been observed of dogs that began to howl for no reason when their masters found themselves in danger somewhere far away from the dog. You can also find cases where the dog does all it can to bring help when its master is in danger of dying.

In the same spirit Rupert Sheldrake and Pamela Smart and others have studied the number of times a dog stood at the window, waiting for its master's return. It was noted that by asking the master to return home at random times during the day, the dog would go to the window, stay there, and wait for the ten minutes preceding its master's arrival. The dog would place itself in a position to greet its master even though it was not the usual time for its master to come home. It was by leaving a camera running inside the home that the researchers were able to bring to light this strange and mysterious behavior. Just as certain animals can detect a spectrum of colors different from ours, would it not also be possible that they have communication tools that we are unaware of today? We still have a lot to learn from animals and their way of communicating without using words.

The Parrot—Damn Good at Telepathy

The only animal that has some ability with words is the parrot. Biologist Rupert Sheldrake carried out studies of telepathy on an African gray parrot in New York. What's unusual about this parrot, N'kisi, is that through training, he acquired the rather astonishing repertoire of 950 words. The test consisted of showing images to the parrot's owner while the owner was in an adjoining room. The images being shown corresponded to words in the parrot's repertoire. In 32 percent of the cases, the parrot succeeded in finding the right image in his vocabulary. This result is statistically very significant.

In the light of these experiments on telepathy, we can confirm that this mysterious form of communication doesn't work all the time and that it seems to work better with certain people rather than others. A little like the case of a radio station that you're looking for while driving on the thruway and you find that sometimes it works and sometimes it cuts out.

Distance Operation of a Robotic Arm Using Thought

Stroke victims who have not regained all their motor functions can now benefit from a new generation of treatment. Using thought it is now possible, for example, to grasp a thermos using an articulated mechanical arm and drink from it using a straw. Neuronal implants pick up specific waves from the brain. These waves are converted to electric impulses in implanted chips and are then transmitted to a computer that is able to move the mechanical arm according to the thoughts and commands of the person. Cerebral implants are surgically placed in regions of the brain known for obeying orders from thoughts. This represents considerable progress for patients since it allows them relative autonomy in using certain simple movements from everyday life, such as drinking a glass of water without help. For a patient who is paralyzed and cannot speak, it represents a big step toward freedom. Twenty years earlier no one could have believed that it would be possible to control an object using thought alone. These experiments cannot be compared to pure telepathy, but the progress opens new avenues toward possible ways of communicating using the brain—ways that are still unknown to us.

THE POWER OF MAGNETISM

A Little History and a Little Biology

In 1820 Hans Christian Oersted, a Danish scientist, successfully conducted an experiment that opened an approach to magnetism. He placed a compass beside a wire that was carrying an electric current. He stopped the current. The direction of the compass needle changed. It was simple but revealing. A compass is made up of a magnetized needle that turns freely on a pivot in order to show the direction of magnetic north on the Earth. This ancestor of the GPS allows you to orient yourself to the four cardinal directions. The experiment is fascinating; nonvisible waves can change the direction of a metal needle. The invisible becomes visible, and this is the beginning of the story. . . .

Magnetism is a physical phenomenon by means of which the forces of attraction or repulsion of an object enter into action on another object or on electric charges in movement. Magnetizable objects can interact with a magnetic field by reacting in their orientation and displacement. When we're speaking about objects that can be made to move with magnets, things are simple. But today a medical discovery has revolutionized the facts of the situation. Researchers at the National Academy of Science have uncovered in the human brain the presence of magnetized particles—magnetite crystals—that connect us to external magnetic fields. These are precisely the same crystals of magnetite that are present in compass needles. Therefore, we are, without knowing it, emitters and receptors. Learning how these emitters-receptors work will allow us to discover an unsuspected power within us, even though we don't know how to use it.

In the past pigeons served as a first study model. They, in fact, have these same metallic particles available in their brains, and they use them to move through the air as if they had invisible radar. It's an effective and robust navigation system that allows them to travel around the planet from one end to the other and through all meridians. During great migrations they use terrestrial electromagnetic fields to orient themselves and find their way.

In humans discoveries about magnetism have led to new solutions for making diagnoses and treating certain diseases. It's a method of healing using nonchemical procedures that are very well tolerated. Scientists are in the process of opening new avenues that could even lead to changing behavior—such as transforming a quiet individual into an aggressive individual, or vice versa. It's easy to understand the limits of these new treatments, which should not be put into just anyone's hands. Prescribed and applied by doctors, there are minimal risks, but in the hands of dictators, their development could be a disaster.

Therapeutic Uses of Magnetism

Magnetism is prescribed in the case of migraines and for the treatment of depression, to give only two examples. Let's come back to popular beliefs about magnetism. It has always been the case that in the countryside you could hear talk of the strange and mysterious powers of healers or magnetizers, and country folk would secretly pass around their whereabouts. Everyone knows what these people do, and everyone knows that one day they might have to consult one. There is no serious study that shows the effectiveness of these treatments. And yet you can always find people who will tell you stories of miraculous cures that they conducted or witnessed. Usually it's a question of illnesses for which traditional medicine has failed and can offer nothing to either cure or comfort the patients.

In my career as a doctor, I have witnessed multiple examples: warts, migraines, rheumatic pain, asthma . . . the list is long. Each time I have to acknowledge my perplexity and my embarrassment, and I have always categorized these cures under the heading of placebo effect.

The Placebo Effect

The placebo effect happens when a doctor prescribes pills containing nothing but sugar, for example, and explains to the patient that it is a very effective treatment for treating some symptom—such as pain or insomnia. One-third of the patients will find the medication effective and even more so when the doctor has vigorously reminded them not to exceed the prescribed dosage. The principle is based on the strong belief that a given medicine can cure. It happens for about 30 percent of the people, even if the medication contains nothing at all. This realization, by the way, obliges the pharmaceutical industry to always test a new medication against a placebo to ensure that the beneficial effect does not depend only on the placebo effect.

Depression

One person in five will be struck with nervous depression during his life. This is a figure that shows to what extent this phenomenon is significant in our society. It is not a question of a passing state of mind but a real disease that destroys the lives of those struck down by it, sometimes even leading to suicide. Depression can manifest in different ways, which makes its diagnosis tricky. In classic cases the subject feels an immense sadness, a loss of motivation—even for simple things—and the notion that as an individual, his self-worth has plummeted. In other cases it can appear as excessive fatigue, a loss of appetite or episodes of bulimia, difficulties concentrating and making decisions, a decrease in libido, a strong irritability or aggressiveness, or a sharp decrease in feeling pleasure. I attach particular importance to hidden depression. No one can detect what is happening. The subjects themselves would not even think for an instant they have been struck by a real depression.

The body throws out calls for help, very often without the person or those around him being able to hear these calls of distress. It's a disease with no voice that very quietly develops and causes more and more damage every day.

Risk factors can be associated with depression. It has been noted that in certain cases the serotonin level (a neurotransmitter that is essential to the central nervous system) weakens. Hypothyroidism or menopause can, through the hormonal changes that they induce, contribute to a state of depression or set it off. Stress is also a known cause, especially when it continues over too long a period. The season also plays a role. There are seasonal depressions that manifest in autumn and winter known under the acronym of SAD (seasonal affective disorder). They can be treated very effectively with a therapy that uses light. Finally, it can happen that depression is easily explained by the advent of brutal exterior events such as a divorce, a death, or the loss of a job. The disease then appears as a way of reacting to the situation.

In treating depression today there is an extensive therapeutic arsenal, but it does not always manage to completely heal the person who is suffering. Psychotherapy or psychoanalysis can help by searching deeply into particular events in the past that could explain the depression. Sigmund Freud opened numerous avenues to penetrate deeply into the unconscious and understand the roots of certain depressions. There are numerous medications that attempt to improve mood, but the results remain uneven. Also, the risk of addiction exists and should not be ignored.

Recently, a new treatment technique for depression has appeared and is giving promising results, allowing patients to be cured or have their state significantly improved—without medication, without risk, and without side effects. The new technique is called transcranial magnetic stimulation. The person is placed in a seated position. The doctors use a large magnet situated above the person's head that produces a magnetic field for about ten minutes. This technique allows a precise region of the brain to be activated through stimulation from the electromagnetic rays. The particular region of the brain targeted is known to be active in the regulation of emotions, joy, and pleasure. This little region is situated 1.6 cm (0.6 inches) below the scalp in the left lateral prefrontal cortex. In order to properly locate this region, which is the size of a coin, the doctors use a kind of cerebral GPS that permits great precision. Incidentally, when the region is stimulated, it produces a reflex contraction in the right thumb, as if to say, "All is well!"

In animals the stimulation of this region has allowed us to better understand the beneficial effect of this technique on depression. The release of dopamine, known for its positive effect on desire and pleasure, has been observed in this method, which is already in use in the United States and is having positive results for many patients. It is a gentle and effective new way to manage a disease that is still creating too much damage.

Migraines and Neurological Diseases

Migraines affect three times more women than men. They are headaches that take place with a frequency and a recurrence rate that varies a great deal from one person to the next. Often, the subject feels the crisis coming on through small neurological warning signals. It also happens that the person, having gone through a number of crises, is able to identify triggering events such as the ingestion of certain foods like coffee or chocolate, an excess of stress, or periods in the menstrual cycle. Migraines are painful and do not always respond to the various treatments offered. The therapeutic repertoire of medications is quite varied, from beta-blockers to Botox, from aspirin to acetaminophen, each one attempting to find something that might relieve or shorten the crisis.

In this case as well, electromagnetic stimulation has given positive results with a certain number of subjects. The noninvasive and painless method is a significant plus factor, especially for those who have been suffering for their whole lives. In a good number of cases, the magnetic stimulation results in a raising of the threshold above which the crisis is triggered, and it has the effect of significantly reducing the frequency of the crises.

Electromagnetic stimulation has been used with success in other pathologies. With chronic neuropathic pain that has resisted all treatment, this technique has produced numerous positive results. As well, with Parkinson's disease, which is characterized by a passive trembling and hypertonia, it has allowed a partial recuperation of motor function. In the case of dystonia (such as, for example, writer's cramp), this method has also proved to be beneficial. At the moment we are right at the beginning of the exploitation of this new therapeutic method, which takes us somewhat off the beaten path. However, the first results are very promising, and they are leading us to consider using this new method in cases that are resistant to classic treatment.

POWERS WE DON'T UNDERSTAND

In becoming a top researcher, the first rule before all others is never to have any preconceived ideas. You need to observe and ponder without having decided anything in advance. Let's take the example of medicinal plants. They have been used for centuries in Africa, in India, and in Asia. From time immemorial generations of men and women have been helped by these treatments without anyone ever knowing the reasons why. For many years now the pharmaceutical industry has delved into healing plants to discover their secrets and to demonstrate or disprove their real effectiveness. For now some ancestral practices have been shown to be useful in curing certain diseases. Without knowing why our ancestors instinctively established a connection between a plant and an illness. In other cases the results were totally disappointing. This research is still continuing today. It is from a similar angle that I have tried to understand if there is a scientific reality underlying the practices of parapsychology. In starting out I simply tried to understand whether these old methods that have been around certainly for thousands of years had any legitimacy at all.

Predicting Your Future: Reading Palms

Palmistry, or chiromancy, has been used in China and India for five thousand years. For initiates in this discipline, the objective is to interpret the pattern of the lines in the palm of the hand in order to establish links with the personality and the person's future. In palmistry there are several lines: the line of life would be the most important, indicating the course of the life with breaks in the line showing disturbances. Chiromancers divide the length of the line into proportional segments in order to predict the moment when these disturbances will occur. This line begins between the thumb and index finger and ends at the mount of Venus situated at the base of the thumb. The second line, the one in the middle, is the head line and corresponds to mental ability. The line of the heart provides indications about your love life. There are also lines of destiny and good fortune. Is there a scientific reality in these practices, or is it entirely charlatanism?

Several scientific teams have collaborated in this research. Dr. Paul Newrick in Great Britain studied the relationship between the life line and the actual longevity of individuals. His method was particularly effective: taking one hundred autopsies he compared the length of the line of life with the person's death date. Contrary to all expectations he did establish a link between the two. The study was conducted on sixty-three men and thirty-seven women ranging in age from 27 to 105. Newrick carefully measured the length of each individual's life line, taking care each time to place the open hand in exactly the same position. He noticed that the correlations were stronger with the right hand than with the left hand. It is clear that a sample of one hundred individuals is a first approach and that it would be necessary to carry out research on larger numbers of people in order to verify these first results. Other studies have been conducted along these lines. As an example, I will mention a recent study undertaken by Dr. N. Madan in India, which was conducted on 336 children aged three to six. He was able to establish a link between the appearance of dental caries and the configuration in prints of the third finger of the hand.

If we make a correlation between the appearance of wrinkles and the duration of life, it has been established by scientific studies that when you look ten years younger, you live ten years longer. As an illustration of such studies, you need only consider how smoking really speeds up the formation of wrinkles on the face, makes the complexion gray, and sharply diminishes life expectancy through the early appearance of cardiovascular disease and cancer. Without having recourse to palmistry, there are other means for predicting life expectancy. All you need to do is to observe how quickly an elderly person walks in order to predict that person's life expectancy.

Dr. Rachel Cooper studied other indicators for objectively predicting life expectancy without using a crystal ball. Studying elderly individuals she found clear links between life expectancy and a number of physical parameters such as the strength of one's handshake, walking speed, and how fast one rose from a chair. In general, the more an individual moves around quickly, the more good muscular strength is maintained and the more life expectancy is extended.

Show Me Your Hands

Hands often tell the story of one's life. In the hands of the hardworking laborer and in the hands of the pianist, much is written. Hands reveal a person's age more reliably than the face. When we think of using sunscreen lotion to protect the face, we should also have the same reflex for the hands, which are very exposed to the sun.

The Length of the Index Finger and Prostate Cancer

A recent British study has shown that the length of the index finger is a predictive factor in prostate cancer. If a man is less than sixty years old and his index finger is longer than his ring finger, the risk that he will develop prostate cancer falls by 87 percent. If the man is more than 60 years old, the risk falls by 33 percent. It also turns out that the length of the index finger is related to the hormone level during pregnancy. In practice, the less boys are exposed to testosterone, the longer the index finger will be, thus increasing their protection against prostate cancer.

What Our Nails Tell Us

Certain pathologies show up in the appearance of our hands—in particular in our nails. Here are some examples.

- The formation of Hippocratic fingers (nail clubbing) is a sign that must always be taken very seriously, because it is a strong signal of serious disease such as lung cancer. It shows up as nails that are slightly humped like the glass on a wristwatch. The nail increases in convexity in two directions—width and height. The consistency of the nail remains normal, but its shape changes.
- The color of the nails is also an important indicator: if they take on a violet tinge, you should immediately consult a doctor. This color called *cyanosis* means that the blood is not sufficiently oxygenated. There can be a number of possible causes: breathing deficiencies linked to chronic lung disease, lung cancer, or cardiovascular disease in which the heart is no longer pumping as it should. In order to confirm this suspicion, you should also check the color of the lips. If they also have a violet tinge, the diagnosis is confirmed. In contrast, white spots under the nails do not indicate any particular health risk.

Handwriting Analysis: A Way of Diagnosing Illnesses

Graphology is used to try to understand a person's psychological characteristics based on an analysis of handwriting. Certain recruiting offices use this technique in order to try to do a better job of sizing up an individual before possible placement. The issue here is knowing whether, based on a writing sample, you would be able to detect the appearance of certain diseases and if graphology would prove to be a reliable technique for determining the personality and psychology of an individual. We should note, however, that it is becoming easier today to find a person's genetic code from a single hair (of which we lose at least fifty a day) than by analyzing a writing sample. Besides, no intimate information filters through in text messages and e-mails. And finally, it is clear that a person suffering from Parkinson's disease will have his trembling show up in his handwriting.

However, there is one study of handwriting that stands out. It was conducted by Dr. Stéphane Mouly at the Lariboisière Hospital in France. Her study showed that graphology can be used to determine if individuals show any risk of suicide. The authors of this study chose forty subjects who had carried out an attempt at suicide and a group of forty individuals who showed no predetermined psychological risk. The eighty letters analyzed showed that in the suicide group there were characteristic differences compared to the control group. It should be mentioned as well that graphology is also used in a legal context to authenticate an official text such as a will, which shows that there are serious criteria in the analysis of handwriting.

THE SENSE OF OBSERVATION

You need only observe a person's face and body in order to have a general idea of her state of health, before even looking at her hands.

Does a Person's Height Increase the Risk of Cancer?

By studying more than a million women in Great Britain, researchers at the University of Oxford have shown that height can be connected to the risk of cancer, regardless of the type of cancer. The results showed that the taller a woman was, the greater was her risk of cancer. When a woman's height is more than 1.73 meters (68 inches), her risk of developing cancer increases by 37 percent compared to a woman who measures less than 1.50 meters (59 inches). Above this height the risk of cancer increases by 16 percent every 10 centimeters (4 inches).

Another study conducted by a team of researchers at the Yale School of Public Health has shown that the taller a man is, the greater his risk of developing testicular cancer. The researchers discovered that above 1.80 meters (70.8 inches), the risk of testicular cancer increases by 13 percent every 5 centimeters (2 inches).

A Good Distribution of Fat Improves Your Protection

It's better to look like a pear than an apple. Distribution of fat is a good indicator of cardiovascular risk. When the fat is situated around the waist and the stomach, the cardiovascular risks are higher than when the excess fat is below the belt. A scientific study has even shown that women with big bottoms enjoyed a cardiovascular protection factor. In order to have a very rough idea of your own risk, if your waist is more than 80 centimeters (31 inches) for women and more than 94 centimeters (37 inches) for men, consult your doctor. It is important to detect as quickly as possible what is defined in medicine as the metabolic syndrome. Three criteria among the following indicate limits that should not be exceeded: a waist measurement of 31 inches for women and 37 inches for men, triglycerides in the blood above 1.50 g/l, arterial pressure above 130/85 mm Hg, a level of good cholesterol that is too low, a level of bad cholesterol that is too high, and a glycemic index above 1 g/l. If the diagnosis shows an excess in three of these indicators, the door is open for a bonfire of cardiovascular disease.

THE STARS

Are We Conditioned by the Month in Which We Were Born?

There are numerous magazines that offer a horoscope column, and let's be honest, there are many of us who read it, even if we don't believe in it. But whether it's lunar or solar, is there really something you can trust in these predictions? Of course, if you try reading the horoscope of some other astrological sign instead of your own horoscope, you will likely find details that relate to you as well. Sometimes you will notice coincidences between the astrological predictions and events in your week. In order to clarify this subject, scientific teams have studied the links that could exist between the birth month and the characteristics of the life of an individual. Such powerful databases exist today on the health of populations of individuals that we can identify links between birth dates and a person's health. We are speaking of course of studies that look back over the life of the individual. The first study was conducted in Vietnam by an Austrian team. It shows that women born in July and August have fewer children. The atmospheric conditions, as well as the type of food consumed during pregnancy can have a possible influence on the reproductive organs of the fetus. It is possible that certain deficiencies play a role. As an example, it was shown that a deficiency of folic acid during pregnancy could be behind the malformation in the fetus called spina bifida. The same researchers studied sample populations in Romania and observed that the fertility of women born in June was higher than those born in December.

In another area Dr. L. Nilsson's team in Sweden researched links between a child's birth month and the risk of allergies. It is true that allergies affect more and more people (see chapter 4). The incidence has doubled in fifteen years. Today one person in three suffers from allergies. The symptoms range from a simple allergic rhinitis up to asthma. All ages are affected. The Swedish study was conducted on 209 children aged twelve to fifteen. The researchers found that children born between September and February had more allergic issues, both in the case of pollen and in the case of food allergies. Conversely, they found that sensitivity to pollen and the resulting allergic rhinitis and conjunctivitis were less frequent in children born in the spring. It is possible that children born during a time when they would be exposed to pollen are better protected against future contact with these allergens. Belgian scientists were interested in the link between Crohn's disease (a disease of chronic intestinal inflammation) and a person's birth month. The study was conducted on 1,025 patients. A significant correlation was uncovered between the birth month and the frequency of this disease. The researchers found a greatly reduced risk of developing this disease in those born in the month of June. Could the amount of sunlight play a protective role in certain diseases? It is clear that exposure to sunlight makes us think of the influence of vitamin D, which is produced from sunlight on the skin, and its role in the prevention of numerous diseases. Dr. H. K. Bayes in Glasgow, Scotland, has researched links that could exist between MS (multiple sclerosis) and the birth month. To do that he studied a sample group in Scotland, which had the highest incidence in the world of MS. The researchers found that in a large sampling of this group, there were links between the birth month and the disease. Children of both sexes born in April had 22 percent more MS than expected, compared to 16 percent less for children born in the autumn. Also in Great Britain another medical team at the University of Oxford researched connections between the birth month and anorexia nervosa. They found a greater frequency in children born between the months of March and June and a lesser frequency in those born between the months of September and October.

Does the Moon Have an Influence?

From the very beginning the moon has given rise to a veritable mythology. It ranges from diseases that appear following the moon's cycle to its link to the birth rate, from temperaments that change following its position to disturbing phenomena that happen during the full moon. Such topics open the door to all kinds of speculation. The arrival of the first men on the lunar surface in 1969 has done little to change the imagination that surrounds this heavenly body. Perhaps what history will retain about this age-old body will be only this first conquest in space. Here too it is interesting to turn to science.

Dr. F. Ahmad's team in Glasgow found, by observing seven thousand patients admitted to the hospital with a stroke, that there was a rise in the frequency of admissions during periods of the full moon. No explanation has been found for this coincidence. As well, Dr. E. M. Roman in Spain researched the influence of the full moon on hospital admissions for bleeding in the digestive tract. He observed a rhythm of admissions of one per day during periods of the full moon and a frequency of about one every other day at other times. Other teams in Iran have highlighted links between renal colic (kidney stones) and lunar cycles. Do changes in lunar cycles influence certain atmospheric conditions that then affect our health? Or for superstitious individuals, does the full moon increase their stress?

Death Happens More Often at Certain Hours

In other areas scientific explanations allow us to finally understand certain observations that until now seemed linked to chance. It has been observed in all countries that the death rate, regardless of the cause, other than traffic accidents, was higher in the early hours of the morning. Certain people attribute this phenomenon to the wish of the dying person to wait for the first rays of the sun before departing.

The explanation stems from a protein secreted under the control of our biological clock. In practice, it involves a gene that acts upon our internal clock and on the contraction of cardiac cells making them more vulnerable at dawn and provoking disturbances in cardiac rhythm for a heart that is in bad shape. In fact, depending on the hour of the day, certain biological parameters vary. For example, plasma cortisol is highest at 8 a.m. Cortisol increases the amount of sugar in the blood, providing energy and muscular strength. These rhythms linked to the hour of the day can shift later (toward 10 or 11 a.m.) or earlier (5 or 6 a.m.). These shifts between individuals help us understand why certain people are morning people and others evening people.

Influence of the Date of Birth on the Date of Death

Professor David Phillips, of the sociology department at the University of California in San Diego, studied the influence of date of birth on death. He began with a very large sample group composed of 2.7 million people. Analyses showed that the mortality rate of women rose significantly in the week following their birthday. The scientist thought that in order to stay the course until a date that was strongly symbolic, women would do all they could to extend their life up to that date, letting go once the date arrived. With men what happens is the reverse—mortality rises in the week before the birth date. For men the birth date seems to be a source of stress.

For the time being we are without rational explanations to understand the extent of all these phenomena, and all we can do is observe them. It is clear that current databases storing various health events of a given person can easily be matched with meteorological data, a birth date, or a lunar cycle. Perhaps we are on the verge of learning a new form of horoscope . . . and nothing will stop certain researchers. This was the case with an American team who decided to study tombstones. They focused on birth dates and death dates of couples. They made an astonishing discovery. They noticed that men who married much younger spouses lived much longer than men who married women the same age as themselves. Perhaps these young spouses became, at the right moment, vigilant and devoted nurses. These findings were confirmed by a German research team at the Max Planck Institute that looked at deaths between 1990 and 2005 in Denmark. They found that a man who married a woman fifteen to seventeen years younger increased his life expectancy by 20 percent. Marrying a woman seven to nine years younger reduced his risk of dying early by 11 percent.

THE MEANING OF VARIOUS COLORS IN THE SKIN

Most of the time, of course, it's not a question of identifying a clear, bright color—that would be too easy. I would say that it's more like a reflected color on the skin. To carefully observe variations in the color of the skin in the light of day is extremely valuable. All you need is to have a mirror at your disposal and someone around as needed to confirm your doubts.

The Color Yellow

Visible on the skin and sometimes on the conjunctiva (roughly, the part that corresponds to the white of the eye), yellow most often signals an SOS transmitted by a liver that is not functioning the way it should. There are numerous causes: viral hepatitis, cancer of the liver or the bile ducts, alcohol poisoning, stones in the gallbladder, or a benign disease called Gilbert's syndrome (a hereditary pathology that causes an elevated level of bilirubin in the blood without leading to any particular symptoms). In all cases observing this condition should be quickly followed by physical and radiographic examination to find the cause and initiate a treatment if necessary.

The Color Gray

Of course, this is the usual complexion of smokers. The blood is less well oxygenated, and the complexion resembles cigarette smoke. Wrinkles appear deeply and precociously because the small blood vessels that carry oxygen to the skin have a smaller diameter, which explains the poor oxygenation of the tissues. Tobacco is a calamity that causes premature aging and exposes you to a higher risk of cancer and cardiovascular disease. Besides tobacco a gray complexion can be seen in other diseases such as Addison's disease, a kind of tuberculosis of the adrenal glands.

The Colors Red, White, or Orange

Aside from sunburn a red complexion can be linked to a number of diseases. Polycythemia corresponds to an overly high number of red blood cells. This high count is dangerous because there is a risk of provoking a stroke. There are other colors that can appear in the face. A pale white in the case of anemia that can be a sign of small hidden loss of blood, such as from a tumor, or an anemia caused by a deficiency in iron or vitamin B_{12}. An orange color can indicate an excess of vitamin A.

In summary, if those around you comment that your complexion has changed, consult your doctor without delay.

SPONTANEOUS HEALING

For a doctor there's no easy way to accept what is not rational. The first time I was confronted with this kind of situation was when I was a young intern in a hospital. At that time, without understanding it, we witnessed the spontaneous healing of a fifty-year-old woman suffering from breast cancer that had metastasized widely. She had been told and knew that she did not have long to live. Since her disease had been discovered in its terminal phase, it was decided at the time not to attempt any treatment, except for pain control medication on demand. And contrary to all expectations, that patient healed her disease in a few months, without anyone ever being able to understand the basis of this mysterious cure.

I later discovered that this was not an isolated case. Spontaneous cures represent one case out of every 100,000 cases of cancer, which is very few but it is still something. In cancer treatment, for a case to be considered a spontaneous cure, one must have a formal diagnosis that has been confirmed with biopsies and definitely no previous treatment such as chemotherapy, radiation, immunotherapy, or surgery. These criteria also explain the rareness of this occurrence, since it is exceptional that a diagnosed case of cancer has not been subjected to treatment.

Certain researchers have become interested in the elements that all these spontaneous cures of cancer have in common. After all this type of reasoning has stood the test of time. Instead of looking for what treatment could cure cancer, the idea is to research how patients have spontaneously cured their cancer. Do they have something in common? What happened in their lives that so dramatically reversed the course of a disastrous fate? For the moment there is no large-scale research program in this direction, and I regret that there isn't. However, some doctors have noted certain points that deserve attention. For example, certain cancers are more numerous in these spontaneous cures such as neuroblastomas, which are cancers in children. It seems that the children concerned had the same genetic variant that could explain the healing. In adults cases of spontaneous cures of cancers of the kidneys and the breast are the ones most often observed. It seems that in all the cases of spontaneous cures of cancer, the point in common was the fact that the healing took place in 90 percent of the cases following a viral infection. In fact, cancerous cells have a deficiency of the protein interferon, which normally is known to protect cells against viruses. These findings contradict earlier connections identified between viruses and cancers. In this regard we could mention the connections between the human papillomavirus and cervical cancer (today there is a vaccine prescribed for young girls after puberty); the virus of viral hepatitis and cancer of the liver; Burkitt's lymphoma and the Epstein-Barr virus. In the case of spontaneous cure, we are encountering the reverse phenomenon; could a virus have the property of changing the course of events and precipitating a cure of cancer? A number of researchers have begun to follow up on this. Australian researchers have begun by using the virus of the common cold. It may seem surprising to use the cold virus to combat cancer, but despite that, several elements have appeared. This research work was initiated by the case of an eight-year-old Ugandan child suffering from cancer (Burkitt's lymphoma) who then contracted measles (caused by a virus) and ended up cured of cancer.

Along the same lines another team is working on the possible links between the herpes virus and cancer. Working under Dr. Timothy

Cripe, chief of the division on Hematology/Oncology and Bone Marrow Transplant at Nationwide Children's Hospital in Columbus, Ohio, the team treated mice suffering from malignant tumors (neuroblastomas) using a weakened version of herpes. Dr. Cripe then tested two kinds of virus. The adenovirus (often associated with the common cold) and a weakened herpes virus (often associated with what we commonly call a cold sore). The herpes virus turned out to be effective in treating the cancer. Only a single injection of this virus was needed in order to heal tumors in the mice. It is clear that we are at the beginning of understanding these mechanisms as we try to explain the spontaneous healing of cancer. We don't have the solution yet—only scattered pieces of a puzzle—pieces that need to be brought together.

LITERATURE

Abel, E. L., and M. L. Kruger. "Age heterogamy and longevity: Evidence from Jewish and Christian cemeteries." *Biodemography and Social Biology* 54(1) (2008): 1–7.

Adachi, N., T. Adachi, M. Kimura, et al. "Demographic and psychological features of déjà vu experiences in a nonclinical Japanese population." *Journal of Nervous and Mental Disease* 191(4) (2003): 242–47.

Adachi, T., N. Adachi, Y. Takekawa, et al. "Déjà vu experiences in patients with schizophrenia." *Comprehensive Psychiatry* 47(5) (2006): 389–93.

Ahmad, F., T. J. Quinn, J. Dawson, and M. Walters. "A link between lunar phase and medically unexplained stroke symptoms: An unearthly influence?" *Journal of Psychosomatic Research* 65(2) (2008): 131–33.

Bayes, H. K., C. J. Weir, and C. O'Leary. "Timing of birth and risk of multiple sclerosis in the Scottish population." *European Neurology* 63(1) (2010): 36–40.

Bluming, A. Z., and J. L. Ziegler. "Regression of Burkitt's lymphoma in association with measles infection." *Lancet* 2(7715) (1971): 105–6.

Brown, A. S. "A review of the déjà vu experience." *Psychological Bulletin* 129(3) (2003): 394–413.

Chi, R. P., and A. W. Snyder. "Brain stimulation enables the solution of an inherently difficult problem." *Neuroscience Letters* 515(2) (2012): 121–24.

Chi, R. P., F. Fregni, and A. W. Snyder. "Visual memory improved by non-invasive brain stimulation." *Brain Research* 1353 (2010): 168–75.

Cleary, A. M., A. S. Brown, B. D. Sawyer, et al. "Familiarity from the configuration of objects in 3-dimentional space and its relation to déjà vu: A virtual reality investigation." *Consciousness and Cognition* 21(2) (2012): 969–75.

Cleary, A. M., A. J. Ryals, and J. S. Nomi. "Can déjà vu result from similarity to a prior experience? Support for the similarity hypothesis of déjà vu." *Psychonomic Bulletin & Review* 16(6) (2009): 1082–88.

Cooper, R., D. Kuh, R. Hardy, et al. "Objectively measured physical capability levels and mortality: Systematic review and meta-analysis." *BMJ* 341 (2010): 4467.

Crumbaugh, J. C., and E. Stockholm. "Validation of graphoanalysis by 'global' or 'holistic' method." *Perceptual and Motor Skills* 44(2) (1977): 403–10.

Dalen, J., B. W. Smith, B. M. Shelley, et al. "Pilot study: Mindful Eating and Living (MEAL); Weight, eating behavior, and psychological outcomes associated with a mindfulness-based intervention for people with obesity." *Complementary Therapies in Medicine* 18(6) (2010): 260–64.

Disanto, G., A. E. Handel, A. E. Para, et al. "Season of birth and anorexia nervosa." *The British Journal of Psychiatry* 198(5) (2011): 404–5.

Fee, E., and T. M. Brown. "The unfulfilled promise of public health: Déjà vu all over again." *Health Affairs* 21(6) (2002): 31–43.

Hadlaczky, G., and J. Westerlund. "Sensitivity to coincidences and paranormal belief." *Perceptual and Motor Skills* 113(3) (2011): 894–908.

Hardy, S. E., S. Perera, Y. F. Roumani, et al. "Improvement in usual gait speed predicts better survival in older adults." *Journal of The American Geriatrics Society* 55(11) (2007): 1727–34.

Huber, S., and M. Fieder. "Perinatal winter conditions affect later reproductive performance in Romanian women: Intra and intergenerational effects." *American Journal of Human Biology* 23(4) (2011): 546–52.

———. "Strong association between birth month and reproductive performance of Vietnamese women." *American Journal of Human Biology* 21(1) (2009): 25–35.

Hurley, D. "Growing list of positive effects of nicotine seen in neurodegenerative disorders." *Neurology Today* 12(2) (2012): 37–38.

Kirschvink, J. L., A. Kobayashi-Kirschvink, and B. J. Woodford. "Magnetite biomineralization in the human brain." *Proceedings of the National Academy of Science* 89(16) (1992): 7683–87.

Lynn, S. J., I. Kirsch, A. Barabasz, et al. "Hypnosis as an empirically supported clinical intervention: The state of the evidence and a look to the future." *International Journal of Clinical and Experimental Hypnosis* 48(2) (2000): 239–59.

Madan, N., A. Rathnam, and N. Bajaj. "Palmistry: A tool for dental caries prediction!" *Indian Journal of Dental Research* 22(2) (2011): 213–18.

Molaee Govarchin Ghalae, H., S. Zare, M. Choopanloo, and R. Rahimian. "The lunar cycle: Effects of full moon on renal colic." *Urology Journal* 8(2) (2011): 137–40.

Morrow, R. L., E. J. Garland, J. M. Wright, et al. "Influence of relative age on diagnosis and treatment of attention-deficit/hyperactivity disorder in children." *Canadian Medical Association Journal* 184(7) (2012): 755–62.

Mouly, S., I. Mahé, K. Champion, et al. "Graphology for the diagnosis of suicide attempts: A blind proof of principle controlled study." *International Journal of Clinical Practice* 61(3) (2007): 411–15.

Newrick, P. G., E. Affie, and R. J. Corrall. "Relationship between longevity and lifeline: A manual study of 100 patients." *Journal of the Royal Society of Medicine* 83(8) (1990): 499–501.

Nilsson, L., B. Björksten, G. Hattevig, et al. "Season of birth as predictor of atopic manifestations." *Archives of Disease in Childhood* 76(4) (1997): 341–44.

Phillips, D. P., C. A. Van Voorhees, and T. E. Ruth. "The birthday: Lifeline or deadline?" *Psychosomatic Medicine* 54(5) (1992): 532–42.

Quik, M., K. O'Leary, C. M. Tanner. "Nicotine and Parkinson's disease: Implications for therapy." *Movement Disorders* 23(12) (2008): 1641–52.

Recordon, E. G., F. J. M. Stratton, and R. Peters. "Some trials in a case of alleged telepathy." *Journal of the Society for Psychical Research* 44 (1968): 390–99.

Rieger, G., and R. C. Savin-Williams. "The eyes have it: Sex and sexual orientation differences in pupil dilatation patterns." *PLos One* 7(8) (2012): e40256.

Román, E. M., G. Soriano, M. Fuentes, et al. "The influence of the full moon on the number of admissions related to gastrointestinal bleeding." *International Journal of Nursing Practice* 10(6) (2004): 292–96.

Ross, G. W., and H. Petrovitch. "Current evidence for neuroprotective effects of nicotine and caffeine against Parkinson's disease." *Drugs & Aging* 18(11) (2011): 797–806.

Schaller, M., G. E. Miller, W. M. Gervais, et al. "Mere visual perception of other people's disease symptoms facilitates a more aggressive immune response." *Psychological Science* 21(5) (2010): 649–52.

Sheldrake, R., and P. Smart. "Testing a return-anticipating dog, Kane." *Anthrozoos: A Multidisciplinary Journal of the Interactions of People and Animals* 13(4) (2000): 203–12.

———. "Testing for telepathy in connection with e-mails." *Perceptual and Motor Skills* 101(3) (2005): 771–86.

Silverstein, R. G., A. C. Brown, H. D. Roth, and W. B. Britton. "Effects of mindfulness training on body awareness to sexual stimuli: Implications for female sexual dysfunction." *Psychosomatic Medicine* 73(9) (2011): 817–25.

Sørensen, H. T., L. Pedersen, B. Nørgard, et al. "Does month of birth affect risk of Crohn's disease in childhood and adolescence?" *BMJ* 323(7318) (2001): 907.

Snyder, A., H. Bahramali, T. Hawker, and D. J. Mitchell. "Savant-like numerosity skills revealed in normal people by magnetic pulses." *Perception* 35(6) (2006): 837–45.

Toulorge, D., S. Guerreiro, A. Hild, et al. "Neuroprotection of midbrain dopamine neurons by nicotine is gated by cytoplasmic Ca2+." *FASEB Journal* 25(8) (2011): 2563–73.

Van Ranst, M., M. Joossens, S. Joossens, et al. "Crohn's disease and month of birth." *Inflammatory Bowel Diseases* 11(6) (2005): 597–99.

Willer, C. J., D. A. Dyment, A. D. Sadovnick, et al. "Timing of birth and risk of multiple sclerosis: Population based study." *BMJ* 330(7483) (2005): 120.

Woodard, F. J. "A phenomenological study of spontaneous spiritual and paranormal experiences in a 21st-century sample of normal people." *Psychological Reports* 110(1) (2012): 73–132.

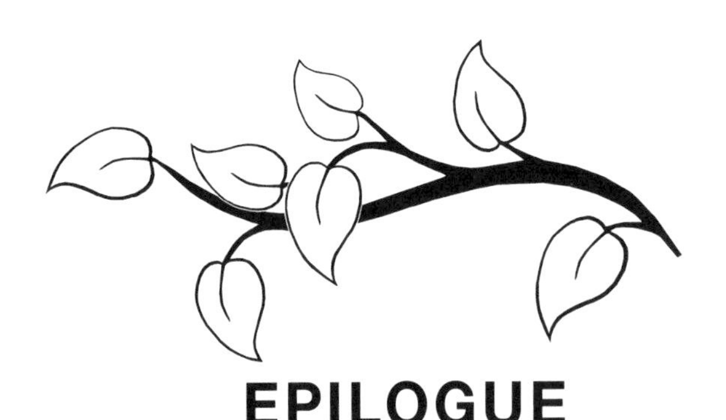

EPILOGUE

We are in possession of immense powers, and we don't even suspect their existence. The brain and the human body hold incredible abilities that we will likely never use, either through ignorance or because we don't know how to discover them, identify them, activate them, and develop them. When a man or a woman succeeds in doing exceptional things, very fast, even impossibly fast, we speak of gifts. This hasty interpretation presumes that everything is set in advance, that some people are born with powers that others don't have, and that it's not worth the trouble to push ourselves because we just don't have the ability. Saying that everything proceeds from gifts that only a few privileged people enjoy amounts to constructing your life from a position of having given up in advance. Discovering one's abilities and putting them into action is one of the most exciting adventures there ever could be. Two thousand years ago Jesus Christ opened a path in this direction with the words, "What have you done with your talent?"

The capacities of the brain and human body open fields of application in extremely varied domains. The brain is an organ that, although it represents only 2 to 3 percent of the weight of the body, consumes more than 20 percent of the daily energy. It integrates and synthesizes functions linked not only to intelligence and reasoning but also to our emotional life and our sense impressions, while storing all of this in a colossal memory bank. In order to have some idea of what a brain can develop into, you need to think of the body of a person who has never done any sports. The muscles are flabby and poorly delineated. After a year of having engaged in athletic activity for an hour a day, emerging muscular forms appear and the body becomes attractive, strong, and powerful. Balance is better, stress less present, and health excellent. The brain too needs to be activated and to do work in order to develop and be as operational as possible. The mastery of cerebral abilities is an essential challenge that will shape emotional, professional, and social success, but more especially happiness.

The big question is knowing in what direction to develop your physical, sensorial, and intellectual abilities. The field of application is so vast that you are in danger of getting lost and spending your life fluttering about without managing to realize your potential. I hope that this book has contributed to giving you a few leads in improving your well-being. To sum things up I would say that there are two fundamental aspects for being in better health.

The first aspect, which I would term essential, concerns all of us, because it is linked to well-being and to health. It is only by maintaining your body and your mind in excellent working order that you can continue to move forward. The old saying, "if you want to travel far, keep your vehicle in good shape" has never been as relevant as it is today. Among the basic mainstays let's mention the quality and quantity of daily food intake and of physical activity. Nutrition is the necessary fuel for life and its quality is in direct relation to our health. As I wrote in the preface, 30 percent fewer calories means 20 percent more life. Poor nutrition does not necessarily kill—instead it makes you sick years later and in doing so spoils your quality of life.

By reading this book you will also have understood that physical activity is the key to good health. Thirty minutes of physical exercise a day reduces by 38 percent the risk of death from cardiovascular disease, cancer, and Alzheimer's disease. Just from this one statistic alone, you can understand to what an extent exercise represents what I call a life duty and an obligation for good health. It's like cleaning your teeth every day—it's not that fascinating a thing to do after every meal.

However, not brushing will end up one day or another causing the loss of teeth that gradually no longer have proper gum support. Maintaining your teeth and maintaining your body means loving and reinforcing a good image of yourself, for yourself but also for others.

The other aspect concerns our particularities as individuals. We are different from one another, which means that our choices in life differ as well. I advise you to regularly set aside a time for reflection, a time to ask yourself what your life would be like if you had the power to make anything happen. A successful adult life is often a child's dream that has come true. We need to keep reaching back to childhood dreams, digging them out from the memory banks, from bodily sensation, daring to speak of all that with oneself, even of what seems totally forbidden by education or by the social milieu. The solution is not always easy to find, but looking for it is the beginning of the path that leads to one's own freedom. Given the difficulty of putting oneself in question, there is a strong temptation to put it off to tomorrow, or to the day after—which means forever. Many adults go through their whole life with the immense timeframe of childhood firmly in mind—a timeframe where you always have time, pushing off toward infinity what ought to be done. You need to be vigilant because in the long run, this strategy will lead to failure.

This book is a first step in opening up the possibilities that are at your disposal so that you can develop the extraordinary powers of your brain and your body—so you can predict, heal, live more intensively, put your well-being in overdrive, and quite simply learn to be happy.

In Chinese medicine it is suggested to those who are ill that they should consult a great doctor for treatment and it is equally strongly suggested to meet regularly with a great teacher or master in order to remain in good health. In reality the great master is oneself. The inner master in each one of us is the generator of perfect harmony. Engaging with oneself in this way is essential to physical and mental development and well-being. And the reason is that we have at our disposal exceptional powers that we are not taking advantage of, or at least taking very little advantage of. There are rich layers stored in the deepest recesses of the individual—powerful resources that are just waiting to be manifested and that are capable of boosting both our physical and intellectual energy so we can go beyond limits that were never before attainable. We all have the potential for self-repair and self-protection against external aggression, but also the potential for rejuvenation and for stepping up to higher speeds of functioning. We just need to move certain levers in order to have at our disposal an effective antiage system and to free up the power that exists within us so that we even manage to live several lives in one lifetime. The enormous medical progress that we are going to find available in the coming years is all based on the same principle: learn to be your own care provider. It is our own cells that will become our medication to prevent disease, cure what is incurable today, regenerate our bodies, and defy time.

Some animals enjoy exceptional powers. Like us, they are living organisms with cells that, every day, perpetuate the miracle of life. These living beings are not made of steel but are made up of fragile tissues just like humans. And yet. . . .

Imagine living to the age of four hundred. That's an everyday thing for a creature called *Arctica islandica.* Not long ago a team of scientists discovered this creature off the coast of Iceland. It looks like a big clam. The number of stria (surface lines or grooves) on its shell means that its age can be determined with precision. Every year a new line appears, just as in the trunk of a tree. For the oldest specimen of this kind of clam, 410 lines have been counted. Perhaps it could have lived longer, but removing it from the sea depths caused its death. If we make some calculations, this mollusk was born in 1601, under the reign of Louis XIII, at a time when the sea depths were less polluted than they are today and were home to different flora and fauna. It's a veritable treasure to have encountered this type of living being because it is a real marker of undersea life over a number of centuries.

The longevity of the *Arctica islandica* is an enigma. How could living cells continue for such a long time without signs of biological deterioration? All living beings are made up of cells that have a number of characteristics in common. They have a gene pool situated in the nucleus, membranes that protect them and permit substance exchange, as well as mechanisms for producing energy and eliminating waste. They are really like little factories, working nonstop all year long, 24-7. How long does a car last today? And moreover it is made of steel and not fragile biological tissue. How many cars would be able to be driven every day for even the short span of fifty years? By studying the cells of this little animal that lives for centuries, we have at our disposal a model for understanding how living cells can resist time and remain in good health.

A team of researchers at the University Hospital Center in Brest, France, have in fact used the heart cells of the clam as a model for studying the impact of toxins in the sea. They are proving to be a very good indicator in understanding a number of biological phenomena. The first point is to concentrate on the clam's makeup. This is all the more easy to do because they are eaten regularly by lots of clam lovers. They are an excellent source of protein with a low level of lipids. Its composition is low in saturated fatty acids, and it contains our famous omega-3s, well known for their prevention of cardiovascular disease. Omega-3s also have the effect of promoting blood thinning, somewhat as aspirin does in other ways. Clams are also an important source of iron (four times more than in the same portion of veal liver). Iron assists in the transfer of oxygen in the cells and participates in the formation of red blood cells. This iron is from a good organic source and is highly absorbable. From only 100 grams (3.5 ounces) of clam, you satisfy your daily requirement for iron. Eating clams allows you to increase your intake of iron in a natural way. Besides iron they also contain a number of other minerals such as zinc, phosphorus, copper, manganese, and selenium. The phosphorus that is contained in the clam is useful in the growth and regeneration of tissue. It is also an important constituent of cellular membranes. Among other things zinc contributes to the quality of immune response, the healing of wounds, and the synthesis of insulin. Copper contributes to building collagens, and selenium helps in the prevention of free radicals. However, eating clams such as the *Arctica islandica* every day doesn't mean you will live to four hundred! It's a pity—we're not going to resolve the question of immortality by using our forks. Still, the study of the clam's mechanisms of biological protection may allow us to understand its exceptional longevity.

Researchers came up with the idea of comparing two types of clams: *Arctica islandica* and another species with a short life, *Mercenaria mercenaria*. As in the game called spot the difference, it's a question of finding the differences that exist between the two, even though their external appearance is very similar. Day after day the scientists explored the biological defense systems that allow the *Arctica islandica* to defy time. What came to light was an extreme resistance to oxidizing stress (thought to alter cellular functioning over time), evidence of highly effective systems of cell repair, and the elimination of free radicals. This clam, given the name of Ming by many researchers, has not yet offered up all its secrets. The grooves in its shell show its age, a little like the grooves of old vinyl records, telling us a four hundred-year-old story.

Arctica islandica lives in cold water, and the cold is a known factor that slows down aging. Experiments with mice have shown that by lowering the temperature of the animal by only 0.5 degrees, you increase its projected lifespan by 15 percent. The cold supports economies in the metabolism. It seems to be an element that might contribute to longevity. But it is only one piece of the puzzle that, once it is put together, will allow us to make giant steps in understanding longevity.

It is clear that a human is not a clam, and clams are extremely different from us. However, both are living and fragile organic beings that carry in their biological cells the same fundamental principles of life. Cells that function uninterruptedly allow life to exist. The extremely fragile cells of this little animal are able to hold out in salt water for four hundred years, meaning they do better than the iron hull of a sunken ship in the ocean depths over the same period. To reach lifetimes of four hundred years, we need to find its secret.

Rana sylvatica (wood frog) is a mysterious frog that lives in the north of Canada and is soon going to be at the origin of considerable advances in the scientific domain. This frog enjoys a considerable power—the power of resurrection! *Rana sylvatica* lives in cold regions. When the ambient temperature falls to 19 degrees Fahrenheit, it freezes and becomes completely preserved. Once frozen it dies. Its heart is stopped, and its brain shows a flat EEG, signaling death. All criteria that characterize the frog's death are present. By the way these are the same criteria that are used in humans in order to provide a death certificate before burial. What researchers from Miami University in Oxford, Ohio, observed in nature, they have reproduced in the laboratory. They froze the frogs. The dead frog in its block of ice can remain in that state for weeks. But at a given moment, when you gradually increase the temperature to return to an ambient heat, something surprising happens: the frog comes back to life. Spontaneously, its heart begins to beat regularly and its brain functions with memory intact as if nothing had happened. No need for electroshock to restart the machine, no specific injection, no extra oxygen supply. How do they do it?

In fact, Canadian researchers from Carleton University in Ottowa observed that at times of intense cold, the frog would burrow into the icy ground spontaneously so it could endure the winter and wait for better weather. In the spring they start out again perfectly normally. Some of these very special frogs were placed in a laboratory so their incredible phenomenon of resurrection could be studied. It was not long before the researchers found a first key. Up until now attempts to preserve an entire living organism have always run into the same problem during cryopreservation. With the cold slivers or needles of ice form and destroy all the cells turning them into a kind of soup. This is why attempts at cryopreservation in animals and in humans always failed in bringing them back to life. But this wood frog found out how. It manufactures its own antifreeze that protects its cells perfectly from destruction by ice needles. And the composition of this antifreeze is incredibly simple: it's a kind of sugar. So, when the temperature goes below freezing, the frog's liver secretes impressive quantities of glycogen that act as an effective antifreeze protection.

This antifreeze spreads through all the organs, the brain, and the arteries and serves to protect against the damage caused by freezing. The frog then has available a powerful weapon to escape the destructive effects of freezing. In parallel to this research, other scientists arrived at the same conclusion that an organic-based antifreeze was essential for assuring effective cryopreservation. An injection of substances composed of derivatives of sugar, among other things, allows cells and organs to be preserved. The research showed that other substances could act equally well to render the freezing more effective. In effect, freezing living tissue has to meet several criteria to be effective. Care must be taken to ensure that the volume of cells is not crushed by the freezing (by manipulating the osmotic nature of the cells), that crystals don't form to destroy the cells, and that everything possible is done to avoid periods of a lack of oxygen, which can seriously damage tissue.

It was once again in studying this famous frog that scientists learned that it produced more urea and other substances such as proline, as well as a specific type of sugar—trehalose. In order to delve further into the mysteries of the *Rana sylvatica*, Dr. Richard E. Lee, Jr., of Miami University discovered that this species of frog was the carrier of a very strange bacteria: *Pseudomonas putida*. By injecting this bacteria into another species of frog that was not able to withstand freezing, he discovered that this other species also became resistant to freezing.

Research is speeding up in understanding how an entire organism can resist freezing and come back to life without any scarring either in the body or in the brain. All parameters have been studied from antifreeze substances to bacteria as well as the time needed to lower the ambient temperature to freezing. In fact, the speed of freezing seems to be a very important factor in the success of the operation. This research is fundamental since it opens new avenues in the preservation of organs that are awaiting transplant operations. Today there is a gap between the number of those waiting for transplants and the number of donors.

The possibility of keeping organs longer in cryopreservation storage (such as what is done now for skin, which can be kept for ten years) could allow us to close this gap. Today, we know very well how to preserve embryos for future implantation as well as spermatozoa, oocytes, and stem cells. In another domain it is important to mention the work of scientists in Japan who succeeded in cloning a mouse that had been kept in a freezer for sixteen years. It seems that the old saying that cold preserves is being verified.

In this context it is interesting to cite the American experiment of the frozen zoo in San Diego. American researchers had the idea of contributing to the biological heritage of humanity and especially for species that are in danger of disappearing. To do that they decided to use cryopreservation to preserve the sperm, oocytes, and certain additional tissue of more than 8,400 animals belonging to 800 different species. It's a kind of present-day Noah's ark that records the body of technical elements specific to each species from its way of life to its DNA. All these animals are living together: polar bears, rhinoceroses, birds, gorillas, and lions. All the means have been assembled to be able one day, with the progress of science, to resuscitate extinct species. Because the zoo is in an area of significant seismic risk, those in charge have taken the precaution of duplicating the samples and storing them in another area that is less at risk.

A few years ago the sheep Dolly showed that the boundaries of the impossible had already been exceeded. In contrast, however, samples taken from poorly preserved mammoths from ten-thousand years ago gave no results at all. It is essential that the cryopreservation be done in conditions of impeccable technology for the result to be a success. The simple example of the preservation of spermatozoids and oocytes clearly shows that exemplary criteria for sampling and preservation are necessary for the success of the operation. It is obvious that the pathway leading to the preservation of cells, tissue, and human organisms is now wide open toward the future, and it is also obvious that in the future this research is going to overturn dogma as well as cultural and social foundations.

The frog has been known since antiquity as a symbol of resurrection. As early as the ancient Greeks, it was considered to be a symbol of fecundity and creativity. The banner of Clovis (first king of the French, fifth century) carried an image of the frog; it represented a spiritual quest for perfection, resurrection, and immortality. Here we have a first signal sent forward from the depths of time by this curious amphibian that early on discovered one of the keys of immortality. The frog of the Canadian woods is a perfect symbol of the colossal progress that we will see in the coming years in the discipline of the conservation of living material using cryopreservation. This area of research had been set aside for a long time since it seemed impossible to return an organism to life, especially with its brain and its memory intact. *Rana sylvatica* shows clearly that the impossible, the unthinkable, is becoming possible. The first attempts in the United States at cryopreservation of entire human organisms after their death came to nothing and will in fact never come to anything. The bodies were put into preservation mode much too late and without taking biological antifreezing elements into account. However, *Rana sylvatica* would lead us to believe that in a not too distant future we might see humans suspended in time. Two-hundred years later, these humans may perhaps return to life thanks to new treatments that would cure the disease to which they had fallen victim. Research on this is underway right now.

The boundaries between life and death and currently between death and life are surpassed a little more every day. In 2012 a team of researchers at the Pasteur Institute in Paris uncovered a disturbing phenomenon. The scientists were studying sixteen cadavers, the oldest of which had died at ninety-five. Seventeen days after the moment of death, they recuperated stem cells from muscles tissue and put them into a culture. To the surprise of the doctors, these cells multiplied and differentiated into muscle cells. It is absolutely incredible that cells could revive after such a long period. You need to imagine for a moment what the tissues of a cadaver turn into after seventeen days—a state of putrefaction, an infected hostile environment with a kind of brew of cells. In the middle of this magma, some key cells survive, such as stem cells that have the ability to reconstruct any organ at all. We are beginning to realize that these cells accomplish an amazing feat by remaining alive inside a dead organism that is in a state of decomposition. In fact, they put themselves literally in standby mode in order to save as much energy as possible. In order to do that, they reduce the activity of their mitochondria, which are cells that work as veritable energy factories. The lack of oxygen even seems to help them survive because stem cells in muscles in a state of oxygen deficiency resist better than those exposed to the general environment. In fact, these cells hit several key points: they adapt perfectly to a terrifying environment in the organic world while at the same time keeping their biological potential untouched. It is truly surprising that living cells can be reborn from a cadaver more than a couple of weeks old. This opens immense perspectives, one of which is an ethical source of stem cells that we could never have even dreamt about.

In practice, in order to resist an extremely violent aggression such as death, the cells invent an innovative strategy. They have to stand up to an assault of destructive enzymes, viruses, devastating bacteria, and a severe lack of oxygen. To do that they put themselves into a state of energy fasting, reducing to a minimum the quantities of energy that they use, even though that means closing down the majority of their energy production centers represented by the mitochondria. In this way they withstand the drastic reduction in oxygen as well as chemical and biological attack. They manage their crisis in their own way making a sharp break in any outlay of energy while concentrating on their survival. Today we are right at the beginning of the study of this phenomenon, which would have been considered supernatural just a few years ago. Here we have a path toward resurrection that is opened using energy fasting that allows the cells to go beyond a limit that seemed unsurpassable.

Immunotherapy represents the symbol of a new, natural medicine that restabilizes unbalanced physiological equilibriums. This medicine has us completely rethink the foundations of medicine and has us use our own resources to take care of ourselves. Of course, this new avenue of ultrapersonal treatment is hard to propose to great numbers of people. This perspective has already been foreseen with the arrival of the research on stem cells. Such research represents the pivot point of regenerative medicine that tomorrow will allow us to re-create in the laboratory, the replacement organ that a patient is going to need, using a stem cell extracted from that same patient. These separate pieces could be fabricated on demand or stockpiled to be used as needed.

The cost of this research is a big obstacle. Still today an African teenager may die from a simple infection for the lack of fifteen dollars to pay for antibiotics. Unfortunately, we put up with this because it takes place far away from us. But tomorrow these inequalities will exist in our own country. The authorities will forbid the practice of this new medicine, just as today they forbid the practice of paternity tests in France. Some people disobey the law and send saliva of the father and of the child to Germany or Great Britain; the result is sent back in the mail. When abortion was illegal in France, young women crossed the Channel to have an abortion. Health does not have any borders, and what is forbidden on one side of the Pyrenees can be allowed on the other side. Except for dictatorships citizens are free in their movement and their choices. The recent example of stockpiles of umbilical cords is particularly eloquent.

In France it is illegal to keep one's own umbilical cord. In the United States companies exist for banking umbilical cord blood. One needs to be aware that the cord is very rich in stem cells, and it is possible that in the future, these cells could be a precious tool in the case of health problems. We are not yet at that stage of research, but why deprive one's children of a possible chance for their future. It is so easy to preserve a cord in liquid nitrogen so that one day it might save lives by becoming a source of replacement cells. Once again it's just a matter of going beyond a current boundary in Europe to find a country where the legislation authorizes this choice. The stem cells that we have inside us will be our best medicine tomorrow for confronting diseases that we don't yet know how to treat. They are the best medication, deeply hidden in our organism and needing only to be activated in order to save us.

It takes a long time to become young.

Pablo Picasso

LITERATURE

Costanzo, J. P., R. E. Lee Jr., and P. H. Lortz. "Glucose concentration regulates freeze tolerance in the wood frog *Rana sylvatica*." *Journal of Experimental Biology* 181 (1993): 245–55.

Ferreira, L. M., and M. A. Mostajo-Radji. "How induced pluripotent stem cells are redefining personalized medicine." *Gene* 520(1) (2013): 1–6.

Ieda, M. "Heart regeneration using reprogramming technology." *Proceedings of the Japan Academy. Series B, Physical and Biological Sciences* 89(3) (2013): 118–28.

Kao, L. S., D. Boone, R. J. Mason, et al. "Antibiotics vs appendectomy for uncomplicated acute appendicitis." *Journal of the American College of Surgeons* 216(3) (2013): 501–5.

Munro, D., and P. U. Blier. "The extreme longevity of *Arctica islandica* is associated with increased peroxidation resistance in mitochondrial membranes." *Aging Cell* 11(5) (2012): 845–55.

Sullivan, K. J., and K. B. Storey. "Environmental stress responsive expression of the gene li16 in *Rana sylvatica,* the freeze tolerant wood frog." *Cryobiology* 64(3) (2012): 192–200.

Ungvari, Z., I. Ridgway, E. E. Philipp, et al. "Extreme longevity is associated with increased resistance to oxidative stress in *Arctica islandica,* the longest-living non-colonial animal." *Journals of Gerontology. Series A, Biological Sciences and Medical Sciences* 66(7) (2011): 741–50.

Zhang, J., and K. B. Storey. "Cell cycle regulation in the freeze tolerant wood frog, *Rana sylvatica*." *Cell Cycle* 11(9) (2012): 1727–42.

ACKNOWLEDGMENTS

I want to thank the following people for their expertise, their wise counsel, and above all for their friendship that accompanied me during the long preparation of this book:

Dr. Michel Aubier
Dr. Frédéric Baud
Mrs. Caroline Bee
Dr. Patrick Berche
Mrs. Lise Boëll, my editor
Dr. Fabrice Bonnet
Dr. François Bricaire
Mr. Richard Ducousset
Dr. Gérald Fain
Dr. Gérard Friedlander
Dr. Serge Hercberg
Dr. Michel Lejoyeux
Dr. Jean François Narbone
Dr. François Olivenne
Mr. Antonin Saldmann
Mrs. Marie Saldmann
Dr. Olivier Spatzierer
Mr. Bernard Werber

INDEX

BOOKS OF RELATED INTEREST

The Acid–Alkaline Diet for Optimum Health
Restore Your Health by Creating pH Balance in Your Diet
by Christopher Vasey, N.D.

Natural Remedies for Inflammation
by Christopher Vasey, N.D.

The Five Tibetans
Five Dynamic Exercises for Health, Energy, and Personal Power
by Christopher S. Kilham

The High Blood Pressure Solution
A Scientifically Proven Program for Preventing Strokes and Heart Disease
by Richard Moore, M.D., Ph.D.

Black Cumin
The Magical Egyptian Herb for Allergies, Asthma, and Immune Disorders
Peter Schleicher, M.D. and Mohamed Saleh, M.D.

Tuning the Human Biofield
Healing with Vibrational Sound Therapy
by Eileen Day McKusick

Himalayan Salt Crystal Lamps
For Healing, Harmony, and Purification
by Clémence Lefèvre

The Science of Getting Rich
Attracting Financial Success through Creative Thought
by Wallace D. Wattles

Inner Traditions • Bear & Company
P.O. Box 388
Rochester, VT 05767
1-800-246-8648
www.InnerTraditions.com

Or contact your local bookseller